BRAIN ANEURYSMS AND

VASCULAR MALFORMATIONS

A Guide for Patients and Families

Eric S. Nussbaum, MD

To order additional copies of this book, contact:
Xlibris Corporation
1-888-7-XLIBRIS
www.Xlibris.com
Orders@Xlibris.com

CONTENTS

This work is dedicated to Dr. Charles Drake, a pioneering aneurysm surgeon & personal mentor. To my uncle, Ira Kasoff, a superb aneurysm surgeon in his own right. To my wife Leslie, to my mother, grandmother, and brother. To Nancy Mattsen, Mike Madison, and the patients who've allowed me to participate in their care.

INTRODUCTION

As many as 1 in 20 people harbor a potentially lethal aneurysm or vascular malformation of the brain. What are aneurysms and vascular malformations? How are they diagnosed? How do you fix them? When do they need to be fixed? As modern medicine evolves, more people are finding out they have a brain aneurysm or vascular malformation, and newer, state-of-the-art options for diagnosis and treatment are becoming available. Until now, no comprehensive material has been written specifically for patients with these complex problems to help them make informed decisions about their care. This book is written for patients and family members to help them understand these disorders.

Brain aneurysms and vascular malformations are very serious and complex problems. If you (or someone you care about) have recently been diagnosed with a brain aneurysm or a vascular malformation of the brain, one of the most important things you can do is to find out as much as you can about the problem. The old cliché "knowledge is power" is never more important than in this type of situation.

Until now, disorders of the blood vessels of the brain have been considered so complicated that almost all information about these conditions has been written strictly for doctors. As a result, it has been almost impossible for the average person to find basic and understandable reference material on these topics. The purpose of "Brain Aneurysms and Vascular Malformations: A Guide for Patients and Families" is to demystify, to educate, and to inform. This guide provides a basic explanation of these disorders including a comprehensive discussion of the state-of-the-art methods that have become available for their diagnosis and treatment. Don't be afraid; learn more about the problem and how it can be repaired.

This book is not written for doctors! Although some doctors who don't know much about these problems might enjoy reading it, this book is directed at the average person who is looking for information on brain aneurysms or vascular malformations. Unfortunately, there's no way to get around using some complex medical terms in a book like this. These big and unfamiliar words can be daunting to the reader, therefore, every effort has been made to use simple explanations and analogies whenever possible. In addition, important concepts have been repeated multiple times and restated in different ways to give the reader the best chance to understand some relatively complicated concepts. So if you come across something that doesn't make perfect sense to you, read on. It will probably become clear as you continue. Remember, this is not meant to be complicated; doctors have just made it sound that way.

Finally, it must be emphasized strongly that this book is not meant to represent a substitute for consultation with an experienced cerebrovascular neurosurgeon. These are serious medical problems, and neurosurgeons who specialize in caring for patients with aneurysms and vascular malformations have studied and practiced for many years to understand their treatment. There is no way that a book such as this can cover completely these complicated topics, and individuals with these serious medical conditions should never try to "treat themselves" or decide on a plan of treatment based on the information in this book without the help of an experienced neurosurgeon. Rather, the book is meant to serve as a guide to educate the reader. That way, when you meet with your physician, you can discuss the situation from an informed perspective, better able to understand the problem and the various treatment options that are available. In fact, most of the information contained in the book is exactly the information that I share with patients when they come to my office to discuss treatment options for these conditions.

Please note that a portion of the proceeds from the sale of this book will be donated to research to help cure brain aneurysms and AVMs.

PART I

BRAIN ANEURYSMS

CHAPTER 1

The Basics

What is an Aneurysm?

Most people are a bit intimidated by the subject of brain aneurysms. After all, you'd "have to be a brain surgeon" to figure them out, right? In fact, anyone can understand brain aneurysms as long as they're explained in a simple way. Let's start with a story to illustrate the subject.

Mr. Johnson decides to build a house in the country. He's done very well in the stock market and plans to spare no expense. He buys all the fanciest fixtures and amenities for his new home. There's a single well on his property, and he even builds a small water plant to pump the water to his house. He plans to run an underground pipe from the plant to his home. Of course, the pipe will have to branch a number of times to bring fresh water to all the different areas of his house. Also, he'll have to lay a complementary set of pipes to carry the dirty water back from each part of the house to a main pipe that runs back to the water plant. There the water can be recycled for future use.

Now imagine that Mr. Johnson, like many people building a house, underestimates the total expense of the project. He runs out of money just before he gets around to buying the pipes, and he can only afford soft rubber tubing. Worried about the possibility of a leak, he manages to find a bit of extra cash and buys reinforced tubing with two concentric layers of rubber. Bankrupt, Mr. Johnson has to complete the construction of the house himself. Unfortunately, when Mr. Johnson goes to lay the tubing, he accidentally damages the outer layer of the rubber tubing in one particular spot without noticing. Thinking everything's fine, he goes ahead and finishes the house, putting up the last inner walls of the house that hide the rubber tubing.

At first, everything goes great for Mr. Johnson. He moves into his new country home, and it's everything he's ever dreamed about. He's particularly proud of how well the water system works. He's very happy. This goes on for a few years. But behind the wall where the tubing runs, a problem starts to develop. The area where Mr. Johnson damaged the outer rubber layer develops a small crack. The inner rubber layer isn't as strong as the outer layer, and it starts to bulge out through the defect in the outer layer. Of course, Mr. Johnson doesn't notice anything because the water system still works, and there's no reason to suspect anything's wrong.

Slowly, the inner layer bulges more and more because of the water pressure. Like a balloon being filled with air, the inner rubber layer stretches thinner and thinner. Finally, one day, Mr. Johnson comes home and finds himself knee deep in water. What happened? Obviously, the rubber tubing finally burst, flooding the house with water.

Believe it or not, brain aneurysms are just as simple. If you followed the saga of Mr. Johnson's new home, you'll have no trouble understanding how an aneurysm forms and why it can rupture! Extending our analogy to the human body, the water plant that pumps the water to the house is the heart. The rubber tubing lines that carry the water to all parts of the house are the arteries, and the tubing carrying the dirty water back to the plant are the veins. The area of the tubing that swelled out and then ruptured represents an aneurysm.

In medical terminology, an **aneurysm** is an abnormal dilatation involving the wall of an artery. **Arteries** are thick-walled blood vessels that carry blood pumped from the heart to all parts of the body. They are distinguished from veins which are thinner-walled channels carrying blood back to the heart after the oxygen and other nutrients have been delivered to the body's tissues. Blood flowing in the arteries is under high pressure, while the pressure in the veins is very low. That's why if you cut an artery, you can bleed to death, while a cut in a vein is rarely dangerous. That's also why bleeding from a ruptured aneurysm can be quite serious.

Aneurysms can develop on any artery within the body. Common arteries where aneurysms are found include the aorta, the main artery carrying blood flow from the heart, the popliteal artery which is located behind the knee, and the arteries of the brain. This book is devoted to **brain aneurysms**. As you've probably guessed, these are aneurysms that develop on the arteries supplying blood flow to the brain.

It appears that a brain aneurysm begins as a small thinned-out area on the wall of an artery at the base of the brain (Figure 1). It is possible that the person is born with this area of potential weakness or that the artery is somehow damaged over time, not unlike the rubber tubing in Mr. Johnson's house. Typically, this point of weakness occurs at a branch point where the artery is either giving off a side branch or actually dividing into two smaller arteries, much like a fork in the road. Over time, the blood flowing in the artery pounds against the thinned portion of the wall, and eventually, the wall starts to dilate. Just like a balloon being inflated, the small area of swelling enlarges with time, and an aneurysm is formed. Like the defective rubber tubing in Mr. Johnson's house, as the aneurysm grows, its wall becomes progressively thinner.

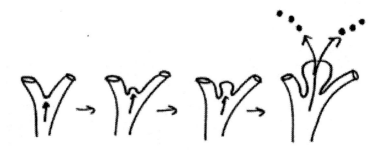

Figure 1. This diagram illustrates the development and eventual rupture of a brain aneurysm. On the left, the blood flow, which is represented by an arrow, stresses an area of "potential" weakness at the branching point of an artery. Over time, this point of weakness dilates into an aneurysm (middle images). The blood can now enter the aneurysm itself. On the far right, blood is actually escaping from a rupture point at the top of the aneurysm.

Why Do Aneurysms Bleed?

Why did Mr. Johnson come home one day to find his house flooded? Eventually, the wall of an aneurysm may become so thin that the force of the blood flowing within the aneurysm can cause the wall to rupture. Imagine a balloon being inflated. If you keep blowing more air into the balloon, the wall will become too thin, and then the balloon will pop. When Mr. Johnson's rubber tubing blew out, water escaped and flooded his house. When an aneurysm ruptures, blood from inside the artery escapes into the space around the brain, the subarachnoid space. For this reason, aneurysm rupture is also called **subarachnoid hemorrhage** or **SAH,** for short. Because an aneurysm involves the wall of an artery, the blood flow inside an aneurysm is under high pressure, and bleeding from an aneurysm can be very dangerous. This will be discussed in detail below.

Why do aneurysms form?

The truth is we don't know for sure why some people develop brain aneurysms. As mentioned already, an aneurysm probably arises at an area where the wall of an artery is thinned out from the start. Most arteries in the body have walls with three layers. The normal arteries in the brain have segments where one of the layers is absent, and this may contribute to the problem. Remember Mr. Johnson's tubing? When the outermost layer is defective, the inner layer can start to bulge out. Also, branch points in arteries where aneurysms usually develop may be intrinsically "weak" sites on the artery wall.

Interestingly, babies and children almost never have aneurysms. Aneurysms can occur in young adults, but they become more common in the fourth and fifth decades. For these reasons, we suspect that a person is born with a predisposition to develop an aneurysm (the thinned-out area on the wall of an artery), and then the aneurysm can grow over time as blood pulses against the wall of the artery.

Most people with brain aneurysms have no identifiable underlying condition or disease that is known to predispose to aneurysm formation. Nevertheless, certain rare diseases are associated with brain aneurysms, and understanding these conditions has given doctors insight into why aneurysms form.

Diseases that result in **high blood pressure (hypertension)** may cause aneurysms to develop by increasing the amount of stress on the walls of arteries. Similarly, if Mr. Johnson had turned up the water pressure to his house, the rubber tubing may have blown out sooner. In addition, people with diseases that affect the structure of **collagen** may be at increased risk for developing aneurysms.

Collagen is a critical building block in the walls of arteries, and an abnormality in the collagen may allow the wall of an artery to dilate into an aneurysm. Examples of diseases which may cause high blood pressure or affect the structure of collagen and are associated with brain aneurysms include Marfan's syndrome, Ehlers Danlos disease, coarctation of the aorta, pseudoxanthoma elasticum, and polycystic kidney disease. **Cigarette smoking** may affect collagen and therefore may be associated with an increased risk of aneurysm formation as well.

How Common are Aneurysms?

Unfortunately, aneurysms are relatively common. After discovering they have an aneurysm, people are always surprised to find out how many of their friends know someone who has been diagnosed with a brain aneurysm. Our best data regarding the incidence of aneurysms in the population comes from autopsy studies. In other words, we have studied how often aneurysms occur by looking for aneurysms in people who've died of other causes. The results depend somewhat on the size cutoff one uses to define an aneurysm, but it appears likely that at least 1 in 100 people have a brain aneurysm. The actual number is probably higher. In fact, up to 5% of people may have at least a tiny brain aneurysm.

Each year, approximately 12 per 100,000 individuals suffer rupture of a brain aneurysm. This means there are about 35,000 aneurysm ruptures per year in North America. It is possible that the number is actually higher, because some people may die from the aneurysm rupture before reaching the hospital, and it may never be recognized that the cause of death was a brain aneurysm. In most cases, the person is assumed to have died of a massive heart attack.

How Dangerous are Aneurysms?

A brain aneurysm is a potentially life-threatening problem. After an aneurysm ruptures, about one-half of people die from the immediate effects of the hemorrhage either before reaching the hospital or within the following few days. In addition, half of the people who survive rupture of a brain aneurysm are left with a significant disability. It is likely that the mortality rate (chance of death) is even higher than we think since many people who suffer from aneurysm rupture may die suddenly and never make it to the hospital. **Once an aneurysm bleeds, there is a great tendency for it to bleed again!** Because the risk of death and disability is so high each time an aneurysm bleeds, treatment of a **ruptured** aneurysm before it can bleed a second time is considered an urgent medical situation. This will be discussed in detail in Chapters 4 and 5.

On the other hand, not all brain aneurysms bleed. We know that many people live a full life, die of natural causes, and their brain aneurysm is discovered only by chance if they happen to have an autopsy for some other reason. So how do we know if a particular aneurysm, **if your aneurysm**, is dangerous? This is not always a simple matter. If an aneurysm bleeds, then it's very dangerous, and it needs to be repaired before it can bleed again. The more difficult question relates to the risk of bleeding from an unruptured aneurysm that is discovered by chance.

What about the person who is being evaluated for some unrelated problem and is found to have an aneurysm that has never bled? In other words, what is the likelihood that a previously **unruptured** aneurysm will bleed? This represents a critical and controversial question. The answer is important because many aneurysms are now being diagnosed before they ever bleed, and a decision has to be made whether or not to repair the aneurysm as a preventative measure. If we had a crystal ball, we could predict which aneurysms would rupture in the future and then repair those aneurysms before they bled. This is not possible with our current technology. As will be discussed in detail below, repairing a brain aneurysm carries some risk. If aneurysms almost never ruptured, it might be more risky to undergo surgery than to leave the aneurysm untreated and take your chances with the small risk that the aneurysm could bleed. Alternatively, if we knew the risk of rupture was high, then treatment before rupture would obviously be the safest option. Unfortunately, the answer is not entirely clear.

For many years we thought that the rate of rupture from a **previously unruptured** aneurysm was about 1–2% per year. In other words, every year, a person with an unruptured aneurysm would have a 1/100 or 2/100 chance of bleeding from the aneurysm. Because these odds would quickly add up against the person with an aneurysm over time, elective surgery to repair an aneurysm was recommended to most people except for the elderly or those with a major illness who were expected to have a very short life expectancy.

More recently, the preliminary results of the International Study on Unruptured Intracranial Aneurysms have suggested that the rupture rates may be much lower than we had thought previously, especially for small aneurysms. Although the data remains controversial and the final results of the study are not yet available, most neurosurgeons are becoming more conservative with recommending prophylactic treatment (preventative treatment prior to rupture) to older individuals or to those people with very challenging aneurysms when treatment itself is likely to result in some degree of injury to the patient. All of this will be reviewed and expanded upon in Chapter 5.

In summary, the management of unruptured aneurysms is difficult because it seems that these aneurysms don't bleed very often, but when they do, it's very bad. Don't forget: **doctors don't always have all the answers either.**

What is a Berry Aneurysm?

In this book, when we talk about an aneurysm, we are typically referring to what is known as a "**saccular**" or "**berry**" aneurysm. These are descriptive terms that are based on the actual appearance of most brain aneurysms. To the naked eye, aneurysms usually resemble a sac or a berry growing on the main trunk of an artery.

There are other types of aneurysms that can occur in the brain. These include mycotic, oncotic, and fusiform aneurysms. These are all rare conditions. Mycotic aneurysms develop when infection within the blood stream settles in an artery of the brain. The wall of the artery can be damaged by the infection, and a small aneurysm can develop. Oncotic aneurysms develop when a tumor in the heart spreads to the arteries of the brain, similarly injuring the wall of an artery in the brain.

Fusiform aneurysms develop when the entire circumference of the wall of an artery is diseased, and the whole artery balloons out. This gives the appearance of a snake that has swallowed an egg (Figure 2). These aneurysms are hard to treat because there is blood flowing through the aneurysm itself to reach the normal blood vessel beyond, and the aneurysm has to be treated in a way that won't stop the blood that is flowing through it. Fusiform aneurysms are much more common in other parts of the body and occur in the brain only rarely. These special aneurysms will not be discussed further.

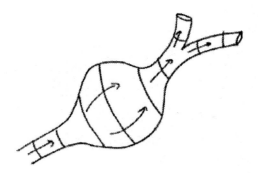

Figure 2. This illustration represents a fusiform aneurysm. Note how the entire artery swells out to become an aneurysm, then narrows down again to become a normal vessel. The blood flows right through the center of the aneurysm to reach the artery beyond. This should be compared with the typical and much more common saccular or berry aneurysm as depicted in Figure 1.

How Large are Brain Aneurysms?

Since the arteries at the base of the brain are themselves tiny, most aneurysms are quite small (less than 1 centimeter or about a half-inch in diameter). Aneurysms may be classified based on their maximal diameter as small (less than a half inch), large (one-half to one inch), and giant (larger than an inch). The size of an aneurysm is important because larger aneurysms appear to have a higher likelihood of bleeding and are also more difficult to treat. Giant aneurysms are rare and very dangerous lesions.

Can One Person Have More than One Aneurysm?

Yes, aneurysms can be multiple. Approximately 20% of individuals who have a brain aneurysm have a second aneurysm as well. People may even have 3 or more aneurysms. We don't know for sure why some people only develop one aneurysm and others develop more. It is possible that some people may have a stronger predisposition for developing aneurysms, and this may occur on a genetic basis. The author has personally cared for a handful of patients with more than six aneurysms and is aware of a single patient with 15 aneurysms.

Just Where in the Brain do Aneurysms Develop?

As mentioned earlier, aneurysms occur on the large arteries at the base of the brain. These arteries are running outside and underneath the brain itself so the aneurysms are typically outside the brain as well. The brain gets its blood supply from the two large carotid arteries in the front and the two smaller vertebral arteries in the back. These four arteries run deep in the neck to reach the base of the skull. They run through the skull to enter the space around the base of the brain (the subarachnoid space). The arteries send branches to join with each other forming a "circle" of interconnecting blood vessels below the brain just inside the skull.

Aneurysms can occur on any artery inside the skull, but they are found most commonly in a few specific locations on this circle where the main arteries send branches to each other. These sites include the carotid artery itself, the anterior communicating artery, the middle cerebral artery, the vertebral artery, or the basilar artery.

Each specific location poses particular challenges to the surgeon, and thus the location is important in terms of decision-making and treatment planning. Some locations are particularly dangerous to treat with surgery such as aneurysms that occur on the basilar artery, and only surgeons with special expertise should take care of people with these lesions. This will also be discussed further below.

CHAPTER 2

Could I Have an Aneurysm?

How Does Someone Find out They have an Aneurysm?

Many people have heard the term "silent killer" used in reference to high blood pressure. The reason is that most people don't know they have high blood pressure until it causes major problems. Unfortunately, the same is true of brain aneurysms. Remember that most aneurysms are very small, typically less than one-half inch in diameter. Therefore, they don't usually cause any symptoms unless and until they bleed. Only the rare giant aneurysm or a very strategically located smaller aneurysm can cause symptoms without bleeding.

Aneurysms may be discovered when they bleed, if they get large enough to put pressure on nearby brain structures, or "by chance" when a person is being evaluated for some other problem. This chapter discusses the ways in which aneurysms are discovered and the special radiology tests that can be used to search for an aneurysm.

Bleeding

Unfortunately, the most common way for a person to find out they have an aneurysm is for the aneurysm to bleed. When an aneurysm ruptures, blood escapes into the space around the brain. This bleeding results in the sudden onset of severe headache associated with neck stiffness, sensitivity to light, and sometimes nausea and vomiting. A severe rupture may cause a seizure or loss of consciousness. Chapter 4 contains a more detailed discussion of what happens when an aneurysm ruptures.

About 1/3 of people will have a mild "warning leak" from an aneurysm before suffering a major rupture. Even a small leak from an aneurysm causes a severe headache, and most people go to the hospital or at least to their family doctor because of the unusual nature of the headache. It is critical that the emergency room physician or family doctor properly diagnose a minor hemorrhage so the aneurysm can be treated prior to a major, life-threatening rupture. This is also discussed in Chapter 4.

Headaches

Most people have occasional headaches. Obviously most headaches are entirely benign, in other words, they don't indicate a serious underlying problem. In fact, the vast majority of headaches are related to muscle tension, migraine, or sinus disorders. Headaches are incredibly common. Aneurysms are relatively common as well. Therefore, some individuals with headache will, by chance, have a brain aneurysm that is entirely unrelated to their headache. Nevertheless, there are a number of features that may raise a "red flag" suggesting that a particular headache may be due to a potentially serious problem.

It is important to remember that an aneurysm can cause a headache in one of two ways: 1) it can bleed, or 2) it can get large enough to put pressure on the surrounding brain. As already described, aneurysm rupture results in a unique form of headache. This headache comes on suddenly as opposed to most ordinary headaches that build up over minutes to hours. Also the headache is typically severe, usually described as different from any headache the individual has ever experienced. Persons who suffer bleeding from an aneurysm typically come to the hospital describing the **sudden onset of the worst headache of their life.** They may say it hit them like a thunderclap. Neck stiffness is also commonly present.

Obviously, if the headache is associated with confusion, nausea, vomiting, or unconsciousness, something serious should be suspected. All these may occur after aneurysm rupture. Finally, if the headache is accompanied by an enlargement of one of the pupils (the dark area in the center of the eye), the presence of an aneurysm should be suspected.

As mentioned, it is rare for an aneurysm to cause a headache until it bleeds. However, large or giant aneurysms can cause headaches by virtue of their size alone. There is nothing unique about the headache that is caused by a giant aneurysm. Brain tumors, abscesses, giant aneurysms, or any other masses within the skull can cause similar headaches by putting pressure on the surrounding brain. The headaches that result from a mass putting pressure on the brain are often present first thing in the morning, may awaken one from sleep, and can cause early morning vomiting. If these symptoms are present, immediate medical evaluation is appropriate.

Other Symptoms

Rarely, aneurysms can cause problems other than headaches without bleeding. Aneurysms, particularly large and giant ones, can press on the brain or the nerves coming out of the brain. This may result in weakness, numbness, double vision, loss of vision, trouble with speech or comprehension, or seizures. **The most common problem that an expanding aneurysm may cause is the sudden onset of double vision with enlargement of the pupil (central dark area) of the affected eye and drooping of the eyelid.** This comes from direct pressure on the nerve that controls eye movement and pupil size on the affected side. Again, these same symptoms can result from any large mass that is growing inside the skull.

Occasionally, a blood clot can form inside an aneurysm and the blood swirling around in the aneurysm can cause the clot to travel out into a main artery. This can block off a brain artery resulting in a stroke. It should be emphasized that this is a very rare occurrence.

In all of these situations, the doctor knows something is wrong but may not be able to tell whether the problem is an aneurysm or some other mass putting pressure on the brain. The results of sophisticated x-ray testing will reveal an aneurysm as the true culprit in these cases.

Incidental Finding

Because many people are now having MRI scans of the brain for a wide variety of reasons, more aneurysms are being discovered unexpectedly. Most of these individuals have headaches or seizures or some other symptoms that are probably unrelated to their aneurysms. These aneurysms are referred to as **asymptomatic** (not causing symptoms) and **incidental** (found by accident while looking for something else). The management of asymptomatic, incidental aneurysms is discussed in Chapter 5.

What Radiology Tests do you do? Do they Hurt?

The only way to find out for sure whether or not you have an aneurysm is to undergo a special radiology test that gives your doctor a picture of the arteries of your brain. There are three different radiology tests that doctors may order for patients when they suspect a brain aneurysm: **computed tomography (CT) scan, magnetic resonance imaging (MRI), and cerebral angiography.**

When a neurosurgeon wishes to obtain high quality images of the brain itself, the two options are CT or MRI. CT is a noninvasive test. The patient lies in a machine that looks like a big donut, and x-rays are taken in rapid fashion using computer reconstruction to obtain images of the brain. CT is fast and inexpensive. It is the single best x-ray test to show up the blood that escapes at the base of the brain when an aneurysm bleeds. Therefore, when aneurysm rupture is suspected, CT is usually the first x-ray test ordered. CT scanning will not usually show the aneurysm itself; instead, CT just tells us that something (probably an aneurysm) has caused bleeding around the brain.

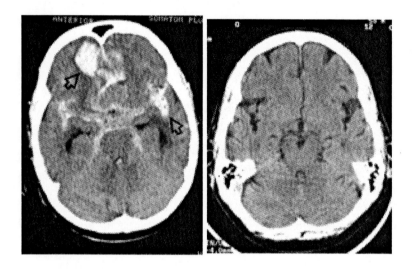

Figure 3A. This is a CT scan of the brain obtained hours after a severe subarachnoid hemorrhage. The white, oval-shaped structure surrounding the outside of the brain is the skull. The brain itself shows up as gray. Open arrows point to white or light-colored collections of blood from the recent aneurysm rupture. The aneurysm itself is not visualized directly by the CT, only the blood that has escaped following the rupture.

Figure 3B. This is a normal CT scan for comparison. The two patients were roughly the same age. Note the white oval outline of the skull and the gray shading of the brain itself. The white collections inside the skull (the bleeding seen in Figure 3A) are conspicuously absent in this normal image.

Most people are familiar with MRI. This is a special radiology test in which the patient lies down in a narrow tube and is slid into a machine that uses a magnetic field to obtain detailed pictures of the brain and its arteries. The most uncomfortable thing about having an MRI is that it may cause a sense of claustrophobia. MRI provides even more detailed images of the structure of the brain than CT. It is more expensive and takes longer to perform than CT, but it does not use x-rays to obtain pictures of the brain. Interestingly, MRI is not a very good test to look for blood from a ruptured aneurysm. MRI is better than CT for detecting the aneurysm itself, but neither of these tests is ideal for identifying definitively a brain aneurysm.

When a CT scan shows that there's been bleeding around the brain or when an MRI suggests the presence of an aneurysm, doctors need a test that provides a close-up picture of the arteries of the brain to search for an aneurysm. The gold standard examination that is used for this purpose is called a cerebral **angiogram**. Angiogram or arteriogram literally means a picture of an artery. This test can be used to look at any artery in the body and is very similar to the test that is used to check the arteries of the heart prior to open heart surgery. The procedure is performed by a neuroradiologist, a radiologist who specializes in interpreting images of the brain, spine, and nerves.

The person is typically awake for the procedure, although slight sedation may be used to make the test more comfortable. The radiologist passes a catheter up through an artery in the groin all the way to the main arteries in the neck that bring blood flow to the brain (the carotid and vertebral arteries). Then the radiologist injects dye into the arteries one at a time while a camera takes multiple, rapid-sequence x-ray pictures of the brain arteries.

As you might expect, an aneurysm shows up as a dilated area on one of the arteries at the base of the brain (Figure 4). A cerebral angiogram to search for a brain aneurysm typically takes about 45 minutes. Most patients tolerate the procedure well. Often, people note a warm sensation or some flushing when the dye is being injected. Some people complain of nausea or vomiting as well. An allergic reaction to the dye is uncommon but can occasionally be a serious problem. Stroke is a rare complication and should occur in fewer than 1.5% of cases. Very rarely, the artery in the groin can be damaged and may require surgical repair. Because these potential complications do exist, angiography is a considered a serious and invasive test that is only ordered in selected settings.

Two alternative, less invasive tests have gained increasing popularity in the evaluation of brain aneurysms. **MRA** is short for **magnetic resonance angiography** and **CTA** for **CT angiography**. Special computer software allows radiologists to use CT or MRI scanning along with an intravenous injection of dye to yield an indirect, reconstructed picture of the arteries of the brain, sort of a "poor man's" angiogram. These are very good screening tools to search for brain aneurysms. They can miss small aneurysms but avoid most of the serious risks of an angiogram because no catheter is actually passed up into the carotid or vertebral arteries. Therefore, we use MRA or CTA to examine the arteries of the brain when we suspect the possibility of an unruptured aneurysm in a patient who has not suffered a hemorrhage. On the other hand, after someone has had bleeding around the brain, it is critical not to miss any aneurysm, even a tiny one. In this setting, an angiogram is almost always requested.

If an aneurysm is identified on MRA or CTA, your doctor may order an angiogram to get a more detailed picture of the aneurysm before recommending a definitive course of treatment. As CTA and MRA improve in quality, it is likely that they will play an even greater role in the diagnosis and management of brain aneurysms, gradually decreasing the need for the more invasive angiogram.

In general, your doctor should discuss in detail with you whatever tests are ordered so that you understand exactly why they are necessary and what risks they carry. Some combination of these tests is almost always required in the evaluation of the patient suspected of harboring a brain aneurysm.

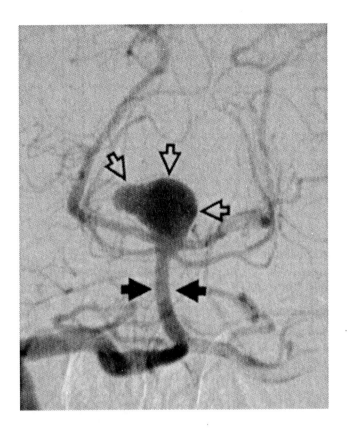

Figure 4. This angiogram demonstrates a large aneurysm at the top or branching point of the basilar artery. Solid black arrows point to the main basilar artery itself, while open arrows surround the large aneurysm. The patient complained of headaches and had a history of cigarette smoking and high blood pressure. One can imagine how the repeated pounding of blood flow against the top of the basilar artery may eventually result in the development and enlargement of the aneurysm (see figure 1, chapter 1 for details).

CHAPTER 3

What are the Treatment Options for an Aneurysm?

Once an aneurysm is found, the obvious question is what should be done about it. Few things create as much fear in the heart and mind of a person as the knowledge that they have a brain aneurysm. Chapter 5 will deal specifically with treatment recommendations for ruptured and unruptured aneurysms, including which aneurysms need to be treated. This chapter discusses the treatment options currently available for a brain aneurysm, while the following chapters focus on when an aneurysm requires treatment and which form of treatment is best.

Observation

The first treatment option for an aneurysm is observation alone. This means that no direct intervention is performed to treat the aneurysm. If observation is recommended, then the neurosurgeon believes that it is safer to do nothing than to embark on a course of treatment. As will be discussed in Chapters 4 and 5, after an aneurysm ruptures, observation is almost never an appropriate option. The risk of the aneurysm rebleeding is simply too high to leave it untreated in almost all cases. Still, in certain patients with aneurysms that have never bled and that are discovered incidentally, observation may be a reasonable option.

If a course of observation is chosen, your neurologist or neurosurgeon may recommend obtaining follow-up MRA or CTA scans in 6 months or 1 year to monitor the aneurysm for signs of growth.

In an elderly patient or in a person with other serious illness resulting in a short life expectancy, it may be reasonable to recommend no treatment and to ask the patient to come back only if they develop new symptoms.

Surgical Treatment

The surgical repair of brain aneurysms has been performed for over 50 years. From a conceptual perspective, aneurysm surgery is simple. A metal clip is applied across the base of the aneurysm so the aneurysm collapses and can no longer fill with blood (Figure 5). From a practical perspective, it is one of the most complex and delicate operations performed today.

The patient is brought to the operating room and placed under general anesthesia; the entire procedure is performed with the patient asleep. Typically, a small amount of hair is shaved from the front part of the head on the side of the aneurysm and the scalp is cleansed with an antiseptic solution. A gently curving incision is then made, beginning just in front of the ear and continuing up and forward just beyond the hairline above the eye. The scalp and muscle beneath are pulled down and forward to expose the underlying skull bone. A window is then cut in the bone with the bone being replaced at the end of the procedure.

The dura mater (Latin for the tough outer covering of the brain) is then opened and the brain is gently elevated to reach the arteries below. The surgeon then uses an operating microscope for magnification to trace the arteries to the area of the aneurysm. Once the aneurysm is in view, it is separated from the surrounding structures by gentle dissection, and a small metal clip (typically made of titanium) that opens and closes like a clothespin is then closed across the base of the aneurysm. With the clip in proper position, blood can no longer flow into the aneurysm, and the aneurysm cannot bleed (Figure 5). The surgeon will often stick a needle into the aneurysm to drain out the small amount of remaining blood. The empty, collapsed sac is left in place and will scar down over time. It should be remembered that the main artery upon which the aneurysm is located is almost always carrying critical blood flow to an important area of the brain. It is essential that the surgeon preserve the blood flow through the main artery and only clip off the aneurysm.

In some hospitals, the surgeon is able to call the radiologist into the operating room to perform another angiogram with the patient still asleep. This is done to prove that the aneurysm is gone and the main arteries are all open and flowing well. If any problem is detected e.g. the aneurysm is not completely clipped or one of the main arteries has been narrowed, the surgeon can fix the problem immediately while the skull is still open. This is a very useful technique and is known as an "intraoperative" angiogram.

After the aneurysm is clipped, the bone is replaced and secured in place with either small metal plates and screws, wire, or suture. The scalp is closed with suture, and a large sterile dressing is typically applied.

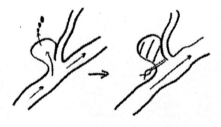

Figure 5. This diagram illustrates the placement of a clip across the base of an aneurysm. Note how blood can flow into the aneurysm before clipping (left) but not with the clip in place (right). After proper clip placement, blood still flows through the main artery and also the side branch artery next to the aneurysm. An improperly placed clip may leave some residual aneurysm or may block the blood flow in the main artery or its side branch.

Aneurysm surgery carries a variety of complications that range from minor, "nuisance-type" problems, to major, life-threatening issues. Potential complications of aneurysm surgery include infection, bleeding during or after the surgery, permanent or transient brain injury, and even death. Brain injury can result in weakness or paralysis of the face, arm, and/or leg, numbness on one side of the body, visual loss, loss of speech or comprehension, memory loss, or coma. The risks that go along with any general anesthesia are also present including difficulties with the heart, lungs, or any other part of the body.

It must be remembered that different aneurysm locations within the brain carry different complication rates. In the majority of cases, the risk of a minor complication should be no higher than 10%, and the risk of a major complication such as a permanent stroke should be below 5%. The risk of death should be around 1%. If an aneurysm is located in the back part of the brain on the basilar artery, these risks may be much higher.

Like most things, aneurysm surgery has both advantages and disadvantages. The main disadvantage of the surgery is that it consists of a major surgical procedure. The complications that can occur are listed above. On the other hand, if the surgery goes well, then the patient almost never has to worry about the aneurysm again. Properly clipped aneurysms almost never grow back, and in most cases, the patient is considered cured. Because open surgery has been around for so long, we have well-established data about its risks, complications, and long-term results.

Of course, it would be naïve to think that all neurosurgeons will have similar results with aneurysm surgery. Different surgeons will have varying degrees of expertise, with some surgeons having a special interest in aneurysm surgery and others performing this type of operation only rarely. In the setting of an unruptured aneurysm, when there is no particular rush to repair the aneurysm, it would be wise to consider finding a surgeon with special expertise in the management of aneurysms.

Endovascular Coiling

A newer treatment option for brain aneurysms is known as "coiling". This is also referred to as endovascular therapy because the treatment is performed from inside (endo) the blood vessel (vascular). Aneurysm coiling, like open surgery, is performed with the patient under general anesthesia. The procedure is performed either by a neurosurgeon or a neuroradiologist (an interventional neuroradiologist) with special training in this technique.

The coiling procedure is performed in a radiology suite. The technique consists of filling the aneurysm from the inside with a long length of fine platinum wire that coils around and around inside the aneurysm. The point is to get the aneurysm to clot off so that it can no longer bleed (Figure 6). The procedure is also referred to as GDC coiling, short for Guglielmi Detachable Coils, the type of coils that are typically used.

In order to coil an aneurysm, the neurosurgeon or neuroradiologist performs an angiogram, passing a fine catheter or tube through the artery in the groin and up to the artery in the neck. Instead of simply injecting dye and taking pictures as with a routine angiogram, the catheter is advanced further into the head and all the way to the aneurysm itself. At this point, while watching on the x-ray monitor, the surgeon passes the fine wire up through the catheter and into the aneurysm. The wire (which starts out in the shape of a coil but is forced into a straight configuration as it passes up the catheter) has internal memory and gradually coils up inside the aneurysm, slowly filling the aneurysm with the metal coils. The surgeon may deposit one or more coils into the aneurysm until the aneurysm is full of wire. The idea is to pack the aneurysm full without having any wire sticking out into the main artery.

Like open surgery, coiling has its own risks and complications. Because the surgeon is working inside the blood vessel, the procedure carries the risk of stroke. In addition, the aneurysm can rupture while the coils are being deposited, and this can be extremely dangerous. Additional risks include the possibility of injury to the artery in the groin. In rare cases, this may require a separate surgery to repair the artery.

The main advantage of coiling is that it avoids an open surgery. This has great appeal to people because it means they don't have to have "open brain surgery". Nevertheless, it is important to remember that other than infection of the brain, coiling carries the same potential for serious complications as open surgery, the same potential for stroke, aneurysm rebleeding during the procedure, and even death. In addition, coiling carries an important additional problem. Coiling of aneurysms has only been used in its present form for about six years. During that time, it has become clear that some aneurysms that are coiled will eventually regrow. It appears that the repeated pulse of blood flow against the metal coils within the aneurysm can gradually compact the coils within the aneurysm forcing the coils out towards the dome of the aneurysm (Figure 6). When this happens, the base of the aneurysm again has blood flowing in it, and the patient is again at risk for bleeding.

Because coiling has only been used for a few years, we don't know the long-term results of this technique. Certainly, the radiologists and surgeons who perform the coiling have gotten better with the technique, and the complication rates have decreased. Also, we have learned that aneurysms in certain locations are not well treated with coiling either because of the high risk of stroke or because of the high risk of aneurysm regrowth. Still, because of the possibility of aneurysm regrowth, patients who are treated with coiling require careful follow-up angiograms to be sure the aneurysm remains fully occluded. Usually, an angiogram is performed 6 months after the procedure and then again at 2 years. We don't know yet whether aneurysms that are still fully coiled at 2 years can ever regrow later on, but it is probably safest to recommend a follow-up angiogram 5 years after the original coiling until more data is available about the stability of coiling over time.

If an aneurysm that has been coiled does grow back, it can be coiled again, it can be clipped with open surgery, or it can be followed over time to see if it grows further. It should be noted that once an aneurysm has been coiled it may be more difficult to go in and clip the aneurysm with an open surgery. The metal coils may prevent the clip from closing the aneurysm off by mechanically keeping the jaws of the clip open. Also, it may be more difficult for the surgeon to collapse and manipulate an aneurysm which is now partially filled with metal wire. The decision to coil an aneurysm, particularly in a young person, should therefore be made only with the input of an experienced surgeon.

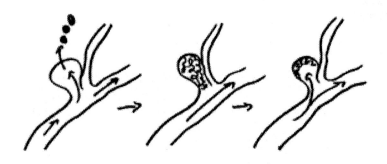

Figure 6. This illustration demonstrates an open aneurysm (left) that is packed completely with coils (center). With the coils in place, blood can no longer flow into the aneurysm, and the person is no longer at risk for aneurysm rupture. Unfortunately, over time, some aneurysms that have been coiled will undergo coil compaction (right). Now blood can again enter the base of the aneurysm, and the person is again at risk for bleeding from the aneurysm.

Deciding Between Therapies

The decision regarding which treatment option to pursue (observation, surgical clipping, or coiling) may be straightforward in some cases and very complex in others. In fact, in some cases, there may not be a "right" answer. The following discussion provides some general guidelines, but it must be emphasized that the final decision regarding treatment should be established with the guidance of a specially trained neurosurgeon with expertise in the management of aneurysms. The overall goal of treatment is to obliterate the aneurysm, preventing any blood from flowing into the aneurysm without causing the patient any disability.

In general, it is appropriate to divide aneurysms into ruptured and unruptured lesions. It should also be noted that an entire separate chapter (Chapter 5) has been devoted to the topic of treatment recommendations for aneurysms.

Except in the rarest of circumstances, a ruptured aneurysm should be treated as soon as possible after it bleeds to prevent it from bleeding again. Therefore, observation alone is almost never appropriate once an aneurysm has bled. There is some variation between different centers, but in the author's practice, a decision is made by an experienced neurosurgeon in consultation with an experienced interventional neuroradiologist regarding which option, clipping or coiling, is most likely to yield a long-term, favorable outcome for the patient.

As a general rule, elderly patients and patients who are in very poor shape because of a severe hemorrhage often do best with coiling. This avoids the rigors of a difficult operation in a patient who might not tolerate the stress of surgery well. On the other hand, young patients and those in good condition are often best served by surgical clipping of the aneurysm. If surgery goes well, the patient is essentially cured of the aneurysm and rarely has to worry about it in the future. It must be remembered that each case is different and unique, and it takes significant expertise to decide on the best treatment option to optimize the outcomes for patients with aneurysms.

Unruptured aneurysms are even more challenging in regard to treatment decision making. Greater detail will be provided in Chapter 5. For now, suffice it so say, that elderly patients with small, unruptured aneurysms probably should not undergo surgery in most situations. Based on our current understanding of untreated aneurysms, these patients are more likely to die of other causes than from aneurysm bleeding. Young patients with unruptured aneurysms are considered candidates for aneurysm treatment, although the final recommendation should come from an experienced neurosurgeon.

Furthermore, the decision between clipping and coiling will depend heavily on the experience and expertise of the neurosurgeon and neuroradiologist involved. Because aneurysms probably bleed less often than we used to think, the most important principle for the surgeon treating the patient with an unruptured aneurysm is to recommend surgery only if he/she feels the surgery can be performed with a very low complication rate. The same is true for coiling.

Special Surgical Techniques

For the sake of completeness, a brief discussion is included of surgical techniques other than clipping in the treatment of brain aneurysms. Currently, clipping remains the ideal treatment for brain aneurysms. Occasionally, an aneurysm may not be suitable for routine clipping because of its shape, because a long segment of the main artery itself is part of the aneurysm, or because the aneurysm is heavily calcified and a clip applied to its neck just won't close. Rarely, an important branch artery emerges from the aneurysm itself and clipping the whole aneurysm will necessarily stop blood flow into the branch resulting in a certain stroke.

In these cases, the surgeon may be able to clip part of the aneurysm and may decide to wrap the remainder with a tough, muslin gauze. Theoretically the gauze reinforces the aneurysm wall and decreases the future risk of bleeding. Sometimes the entire aneurysm is wrapped if no clipping is possible.

In rare cases, the entire segment of the artery upon which the aneurysm arises appears to be diseased and the aneurysm cannot be reconstructed with a clip. An alternate option is to perform a bypass that brings blood flow to the artery beyond the aneurysm, and then to "trap" the segment of the artery upon which the aneurysm is located between clips (Figure 7). This means that blood can no longer reach the aneurysm, while blood flows through the bypass, past the trapped segment of the artery, to reach the brain further downstream.

These surgical techniques, particularly bypass procedures, require significant expertise and should be performed only by vascular neurosurgeons who specialize in this type of surgery.

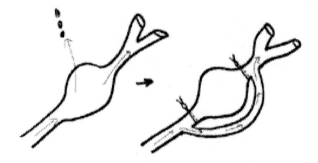

Figure 7. On the left, a fusiform-type aneurysm is illustrated with blood escaping from a small hole in the sidewall of the aneurysm. This type of aneurysm cannot be clipped in simple fashion as in Figure 3. On the right, a bypass graft has been constructed, rerouting blood flow around the aneurysm from the normal artery before the aneurysm to the normal artery downstream from the aneurysm. Clips have been placed on either side of the aneurysm so blood can no longer enter the aneurysm itself. In effect, a bypass has been constructed to carry the blood flow around the diseased or aneurysmal portion of the artery.

CHAPTER 4

What to Expect After an Aneurysm Ruptures

This chapter is devoted to a description of the typical sequence of events that follows rupture of a brain aneurysm. Because there may be significant variation from one case to the next, some differences should be expected in each individual circumstance.

Subarachnoid Hemorrhage (SAH)

When an aneurysm ruptures, blood escapes suddenly from the aneurysm under high pressure into the space around the brain. This space is normally filled with spinal fluid and is called the subarachnoid space because it has a fine lining known as the arachnoid membrane. The bleeding can be minimal, moderate, or severe, and the person's response to the hemorrhage is usually related to the amount of blood that escapes from the aneurysm.

In virtually all cases, SAH causes an immediate headache, neck stiffness, and sensitivity to bright light. This results from the blood mixing with the spinal fluid and irritating the lining of the brain. A common misconception about SAH is that the aneurysm continues to leak continuously until it is repaired. In fact, the aneurysm bleeds for only a few seconds before it stops. If it didn't, the person would rapidly die from the increased pressure inside the head. Usually, a small clot forms at the site of rupture and seals off the tear in the aneurysm. The real risk to the person after the hemorrhage, is that the clot will loosen or break down and the aneurysm will bleed again.

Grading SAH

There are many complex grading schemes that doctors use to assess a patient's condition after SAH. For our purposes, aneurysm rupture can be divided conveniently into mild, moderate, and severe.

After a mild rupture, the person will have a bad headache with some neck stiffness and sensitivity to bright light. The person will almost always seek immediate medical attention and will be acutely aware that something very wrong has happened in their head. A moderate bleed will be characterized by the above findings, but the person will also be confused and drowsy. There may be a brief loss of consciousness, with the person passing out at the time of aneurysm rupture and then waking up with a severe headache and confusion. The patient is sicker and will usually be brought to the hospital by ambulance. Finally, severe hemorrhages produce coma and are associated with a much worse prognosis. These patients are extremely ill and require immediate medical attention and high-level support. They require a breathing tube for mechanical ventilation and intensive care unit monitoring. Severe hemorrhages may cause seizures as well.

Diagnosis

Even after a mild hemorrhage, most patients will know that something is very wrong and will seek medical attention. Initial evaluation typically occurs in the emergency room, and the emergency room physician is usually the first doctor to meet and examine the patient.

The first challenge is to make the proper diagnosis. This is critical because if the proper diagnosis is missed, the person may be sent home and is then at risk for potentially fatal rebleeding from the aneurysm. Because so many people have headaches, the correct diagnosis may not be obvious immediately if the hemorrhage is only mild. Patients with mild or moderate SAH are usually able to tell the doctor about the sudden onset of severe headache, and this history should prompt the ER physician to order a head CT scan. If the patient is in a coma from a severe hemorrhage, then an emergency CT scan is usually obtained and this will show the bleeding. As described in Chapter 2, CT is a non-invasive test in which the patient lies in a "donut-like" machine that takes special x-ray pictures of the brain. It is the best radiology test for detecting bleeding following aneurysm rupture.

In patients with severe or moderate hemorrhage and in most patients with mild hemorrhage, a CT scan will demonstrate the bleeding and the diagnosis is confirmed. In a small number of patients with very mild hemorrhage (less than 5%), the CT may not be able to show up the very small amount of blood that has escaped from the aneurysm. Therefore, if a SAH is suspected and the CT is negative, a spinal tap should be performed because it is very important not to miss a mild hemorrhage that may be the only warning sign prior to a life-threatening hemorrhage.

The patient is asked to lie on his/her side and a fine needle is inserted into the low back region after numbing the skin. This allows the doctor to sample the spinal fluid to look for blood. The spinal fluid is actually produced in the brain and circulates down around the spinal cord. Since aneurysms are located in the subarachnoid space bathed in spinal fluid, even a slight amount of blood spilling into the spinal fluid around the brain will settle in the low back region and will show up on a spinal tap. If the tap shows blood, then the diagnosis of a SAH is made. Of note, if the CT is positive for blood, then no spinal tap is necessary since the diagnosis is already established.

Once the diagnosis of SAH is made, an angiogram is performed to search for an aneurysm as the cause of the bleeding. The details of this procedure are described in Chapter 2. Assuming an aneurysm is found as the source of the bleeding, the patient is typically admitted to the **intensive care unit** or, **ICU**. If no aneurysm is found, refer to the section at the end of this chapter, "Angiogram-negative SAH".

Preoperative Care—Treatment before surgery/coiling

Prior to treatment of the aneurysm, the main goal of care is to minimize the likelihood of aneurysm rebleeding. To this end, it is critical to keep the patient's blood pressure in a normal range (usually below 140) because high blood pressure may increase the risk of rebleeding. This means that the ICU nurse will be monitoring the blood pressure on a regular basis, usually with a special catheter inserted like an "iv" into the artery just above the wrist. Intravenous medication to keep the blood pressure low is often used.

In addition, the patient is typically kept as comfortable as possible in a quiet room under mild sedation. The number of visitors is restricted, and the patient is allowed to rest as much as possible, avoiding active stimulation. The most important thing at this point is to get the aneurysm treated as soon as possible.

Definitive Treatment—Surgery/coiling

The first and foremost danger to the patient who has suffered from aneurysm rupture is that the aneurysm will bleed again. Each time the aneurysm bleeds, there is a high risk for death and disability and the risk of rebleeding is highest in the days and weeks immediately following a rupture. Therefore the primary goal after an aneurysm has bled is to secure the aneurysm in some way so as to prevent rebleeding. The various forms of treatment have been discussed in Chapter 3. The choice of therapy will be further elaborated upon in Chapter 5. In any case, the rule is to treat the aneurysm as soon as possible, almost always within 24 hours after the aneurysm has bled. Whether treatment with surgery or coiling is chosen, early treatment should effectively decrease the risk of rebleeding.

It is worth mentioning that most neurosurgeons will not proceed with surgery to repair an aneurysm at night. Instead, most neurosurgeons will wait until the next day. The surgical repair of an aneurysm is a delicate and dangerous operation, and in most cases it is appropriate to wait until the following day when everyone (including the surgeon, anesthesiologist, and nurses) is fresh and in optimal shape. Under rare emergency circumstances, it may be necessary to operate immediately, even in the middle of the night. This may be the case for aneurysms that have bled repeatedly or when the bleeding produces a large blood clot that is putting significant pressure on the brain resulting in possible irreversible injury if surgery is delayed.

Postoperative Care—Treatment after Surgery/coiling

Once the aneurysm has been treated, either with surgical clipping or with coiling, the patient is returned to the ICU for a variable length of time. At this point a number of problems may threaten the patient and these will be discussed individually. Typically patients with mild hemorrhage will return from surgery or coiling (assuming all went well during the procedure) in good condition. They may stay in the ICU for one or two days and then transfer to a regular hospital room. Patients with moderate hemorrhage will be somewhat sicker and have to stay in the ICU for a longer period of time while they recover. Patients with severe hemorrhage require a prolonged ICU stay, depending on the specifics of their condition.

It should be remembered that the purpose of surgery is to repair the aneurysm to prevent another hemorrhage. Nothing that the surgeon does will likely improve the patient's condition in the short run. Therefore, the family should not expect the patient to return from surgery or coiling in better condition than before the operation. Of course, once the aneurysm is treated, the patient should be protected from bleeding in the future.

Hydrocephalus

Hydrocephalus means "water on the brain" and occurs when the fluid that is normally produced within the brain is not absorbed properly. The spinal fluid (or cerebrospinal fluid) is produced continuously inside the fluid-filled cavities deep within the brain. These are known as the ventricles. This fluid circulates over the surface of the brain and spinal cord and is normally absorbed over the surface of the brain. After an aneurysm ruptures, the blood that escapes from the aneurysm mixes with the spinal fluid and tends to clog up the absorptive pathways for the spinal fluid. This can result in an excess buildup of fluid known as hydrocephalus. As the fluid builds up, there is increased pressure inside the head and, if untreated, this can result in lethargy, coma, or death.

Hydrocephalus can occur within hours after SAH, in which case it can be life-threatening and requires emergency treatment. Typically, the surgeon will drill a small hole in the skull, just behind the hairline, and pass a soft catheter into the fluid-filled spaces in the center of the brain to allow the excess fluid to drain out. The catheter is left in place and attached to a collection bag. This is called a **ventriculostomy** or external ventricular drain. The ventriculostomy is used during surgery to allow the neurosurgeon to drain off the blood and the excess fluid. After SAH, some people will have a permanent problem with reabsorption of the fluid while others will start to absorb the fluid normally again.

You will notice that initially, the fluid in the drainage tubing is bright red due to the fresh bleeding from the aneurysm. Normally, the fluid should be crystal clear, like water. Over time, the fluid will turn darker and become "tea colored" as the blood breaks down. Typically, after surgery, the surgeon will raise the level of the ventriculostomy each day to encourage the fluid to drain naturally on its own. If the patient tolerates this, then the ventriculostomy is clamped off. At this point, the fluid must drain internally. If the patient tolerates having the drain clamped, then a CT scan is obtained to make sure the fluid spaces in the brain are not dilating up from excess fluid. If this looks OK, then the ventriculostomy is removed.

After 1–2 weeks, if the patient still requires drainage of the fluid through the ventriculostomy, then a permanent internal device for drainage of the fluid is necessary. This is known as a **shunt**. This requires a separate operation in which a catheter that passes through a hole in the skull is attached to a long tube that travels under the skin behind the ear, down the neck, over the chest and then into the abdomen. This allows the fluid to drain internally into the space around the stomach and intestine known as the peritoneum. The procedure is therefore called a "ventriculo-peritoneal" or "VP" shunt. This is a permanent device that stays in place for the rest of the person's life. The shunt operation carries a number of risks including bleeding and infection, but these risks are small, particularly in comparison with everything else the patient has been through because of the aneurysm.

Vasospasm

After a SAH, the outside walls of the blood vessels are exposed to the blood that has spilled into the spinal fluid. For reasons that are incompletely understood, this can cause the arteries of the brain to go into spasm (clamp down) any time from 4 to 14 days after the hemorrhage. This may be mild or severe, and in the worst cases, can prevent adequate blood flow from reaching the brain. This can cause a stroke. Unfortunately, we don't have a good way to prevent the spasm from occurring. It is well known that people who've had successful surgery and who've been doing fine otherwise have sometimes developed severe vasospasm and become very sick even days after their operation. We also know that the more severe the initial hemorrhage, i.e. the more blood that escapes during the hemorrhage, the more likely the person is to develop spasm.

When vasospasm does occur, the person may develop increasing headache, confusion or sleepiness. Alternatively, they may develop weakness or paralysis involving one side of the body or both legs. Any unexplained deterioration in function that comes on between four and fourteen days after the initial bleeding may be due to vasospasm, and this must be excluded as a possible cause.

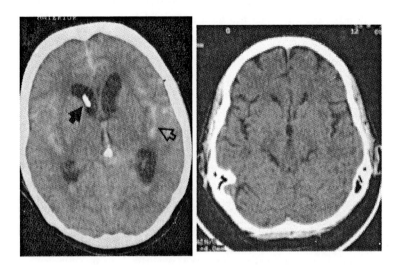

Figure 8A. This CT scan of the brain shows the bright white linear shape of a ventriculostomy tube (black arrow) that has been inserted into the black, fluid-filled ventricles at the center of the brain. The fluid cavities are larger than normal because of impaired absorption of fluid due to the recent hemorrhage. An open arrow points to blood that is layering in the subarachnoid space from a recent aneurysm rupture. The blood appears as white or light-colored material against the gray background of the normal brain. The thick bone of the skull shows up as the white oval shape around the outside of the brain.

Figure 8B. This normal CT scan has been added for comparison. Note the small (normal) size of the dark, fluid-filled ventricles at the center of the brain. Also note the absence of the light-colored areas (the blood) that were present on Figure 8A.

To prevent vasospasm, most people who suffer aneurysm rupture are treated with a medication called nimodipine. This drug has been shown to improve the outcome in patients with vasospasm, although the exact mechanism by which nimodipine achieves this is uncertain. To treat the spasm, patients are kept well hydrated and their blood pressure is kept at a high level. The idea is to keep lots of blood flowing through the arteries to prevent them from clamping down. Of course, if the aneurysm has not been repaired, raising the blood pressure may be dangerous since it may cause the aneurysm to rebleed. Therefore, it is best to have the aneurysm treated either with surgery or with coiling before the vasospasm risk period begins, four days after the SAH.

If these measures don't work to combat the spasm, an angiogram is usually performed to document the degree and location of the spasm. The neuroradiologist can sometimes infuse a medicine called papaverine directly into the narrowed arteries. This may cause the arteries to dilate or open up. At times, the neuroradiologist can even place a small catheter with a balloon on its tip up into the narrowed part of the artery and then inflate the balloon to cause the artery to dilate. This is known as balloon angioplasty. These are sophisticated techniques that should only be performed by specially trained neuroradiologists or neurosurgeons.

Electrolyte Imbalance

After SAH, there is a tendency for the body to temporarily lose the ability to properly regulate the normal salts (electrolytes) in the blood stream. For this reason, the doctor will carefully monitor the salt balance within the blood stream and correct any abnormalities, most commonly a low sodium level. Rarely, electrolyte imbalance can cause significant problems including seizures or coma.

Seizures

After aneurysm rupture, the blood that escapes into the spinal fluid causes irritation of the brain and may result in a seizure. A seizure, also sometimes called an epileptic fit, represents an abnormal discharge of electrical activity within the brain. This can result in generalized firing of nerve cells throughout the brain causing the patient to lose consciousness and shake violently for seconds to minutes. Many neurosurgeons prescribe anti-seizure medications for their patients after aneurysm rupture to decrease the risk of seizure activity. Surgical repair of an aneurysm may further increase the risk of having a seizure because the brain has to be lifted up to reach the aneurysm underneath.

Most seizures are self-limiting i.e. they stop by themselves with or without any intervention. Nevertheless, treatment with medicines to stop a prolonged seizure may be critically important, and patients are observed closely for this after SAH. The anti-seizure medications may be continued for a variable length of time after SAH. Occasionally, patients who actually have seizures after aneurysm rupture may need to remain on these medications for a year or longer. These medicines decrease but do not eliminate the risk of having a seizure. In general, the blood levels of the medicines must be monitored on a regular basis to make sure the dosing is appropriate.

Pulmonary & Cardiac Issues

Following SAH, some individuals will have significant trouble with irregular heart rhythms or problems with the lungs. Therefore, the patient is typically monitored in the intensive care unit for at least a couple of days and sometimes longer to care for these issues. After a severe hemorrhage, the patient is usually not fully conscious and may have a breathing tube in place. It may take days or weeks for the patient to recover from the hemorrhage, and it is best to keep the breathing tube in place until the person is reasonably alert.

If the tube must be left in longer than 2 weeks, the doctor will typically recommend performing a **tracheostomy**. This is a minor surgical procedure that entails making an incision in the front of the neck and inserting a breathing tube directly into the windpipe or trachea. This is a temporary measure, and when the person becomes more alert, the tube is simply removed and the hole in the neck will seal on its own.

Postoperative Angiography

After surgery, the neurosurgeon may recommend a second angiogram for a variety of reasons. As described above, if there is concern for significant vasospasm, an angiogram is often required. Even if everything goes fine, an angiogram is typically performed to be sure the aneurysm has been properly repaired. This can be performed either during the surgery or afterwards. If the aneurysm is still part open, a second surgery may be required, so many surgeons are now performing the angiogram during the operation as described in Chapter 3. If the aneurysm was coiled, then angiography should be performed in delayed fashion as detailed in Chapter 3.

Rehabilitation

Depending on the patient's condition, most individuals who suffer a moderate or severe hemorrhage will require some period of inpatient and outpatient rehabilitation after their acute hospital stay. This means that the person is well enough that they no longer need to be in the hospital for special medical attention, but they may not be well enough to return home right away. Rehabilitation facilities allow the patient to regain independent functioning and build their activity level back up to a reasonable point so they can return home safely.

Rehabilitation is typically heavily individualized based on the patient's condition. Some people require only minor work to get back to normal and others need aggressive reconditioning just to relearn basic functions such as walking, reading, or writing. As a general rule, most patients who suffer a severe hemorrhage will require at least three weeks in the hospital and at least an equivalent length of time (and usually longer) at an inpatient rehabilitation facility.

It may be easiest for family members to think of a SAH much as they would a stroke. Some strokes are mild and require little or no rehabilitation. Moderate strokes like moderate hemorrhages may require limited inpatient rehabilitation followed by a short course of outpatient therapy. Finally severe stroke (and hemorrhage) may necessitate a prolonged inpatient rehabilitation and then significant work as an outpatient to regain independent functioning. In general, most people will experience a very gradual recovery over time.

The patient and family should remember that the brain does recover, but it heals much more slowly than the rest of the body. Recovery can continue for several years after a severe hemorrhage, although the majority of recovery typically occurs by one year with only small further improvement thereafter. The author typically tells patients that by one year after the hemorrhage, most people will have achieved about 90% of their ultimate recovery.

Restrictions After Aneurysm Surgery

One of the most common questions after aneurysm surgery is what the patient can do once they leave the hospital. Following surgery for a ruptured aneurysm, the patient's condition will depend heavily on the severity of the hemorrhage. As mentioned above, patients with moderate or severe hemorrhages will probably require some rehabilitation and may not be able to go home for weeks or even months after the operation. In the case of a mild hemorrhage and in patients who undergo surgery for an unruptured aneurysm, there are few restrictions after surgery.

Most people stay off work for 4 to 6 weeks. If the job is particularly strenuous, this period may have to be extended. Non-vigorous activities such as walking and doing simple work around the house are encouraged as early as possible. Heavy lifting (for example more than fifteen pounds) is usually avoided for the first month as is heavy aerobic exercise. Specific restrictions should be discussed with the neurosurgeon who may vary the recommendations in a given case because of unique issues that may be specific to a particular patient.

Angiogram-Negative SAH

In approximately 10% of cases, the angiogram will fail to show up a source for the bleeding even though there is a clear-cut hemorrhage on the CT scan or based on a spinal tap. There are several possibilities in these cases. First, the angiogram may have missed a small or partially hidden aneurysm. Just after an aneurysm ruptures, there may be some spasm or narrowing of the blood vessels or there may be some clot in the aneurysm. Therefore, if an angiogram is normal immediately after someone has had a definite episode of bleeding around the brain, your doctor will often repeat the angiogram one to two weeks later.

Alternatively, the bleeding may have come from an abnormal collection of arteries and veins within or on the surface of the brain. Treatment for this abnormality which is known as an artery-vein malformation or AVM is an entire topic unto itself and will be discussed in Part II of this book.

Finally, the source of some hemorrhages is never identified, even with one or two repeat angiograms. In these cases, we generally assume that the bleeding may have come from a small vein that ruptured and then sealed itself off.

If no source of bleeding is found, the prognosis is excellent, and it is rare for the patient to ever have further bleeding. Nevertheless, the patient must be reminded that "something" inside their head did bleed—either an artery or a vein. In these cases, we typically restrict the patient's activity for at least one month to allow whatever bled to heal fully. Again, the exact recommendations will vary depending on the specifics of the situation.

CHAPTER 5

Treatment Recommendations for

Ruptured and Unruptured Aneurysms

This chapter presents an overview of the considerations that are involved in recommending a specific course of treatment to the patient with an aneurysm. Much of this information is discussed in Chapters 3 & 4. The management of patients with brain aneurysms is an extremely sophisticated area of medicine, and there is no way to cover every aspect of this complex subject in this book. Rather, this chapter is meant to serve as an overview and a framework so that patients and their families will have some basic understanding of the treatment decision-making process. Finally, it must be emphasized that any decision should be made with the direct assistance of an experienced neurosurgeon who has special expertise in the management of brain aneurysms.

For the purpose of discussion, it is easiest to divide brain aneurysms into ruptured and unruptured lesions. As mentioned in chapter 3, the three treatment options for any aneurysm include observation alone, surgical repair (usually with clipping), or endovascular therapy with coiling.

Ruptured Aneurysms

When an aneurysm bleeds, about 50% of people either don't make it to the hospital or die within the first few days after hospital admission from the after-effects of the hemorrhage. Of those who survive, about 50% are left with permanent disability. The most immediate danger to the patient who has suffered rupture of a brain aneurysm is that the aneurysm will bleed again. The risk of repeat hemorrhage appears to be approximately 25% during the first few weeks after the aneurysm bleeds and 40% over the first 6 months. After a year, the risk of rebleeding falls to roughly 1–2% per year. In other words, the risk of rebleeding is highest immediately after the rupture and falls gradually over time.

It is critical to prevent a ruptured aneurysm from bleeding again because each time the aneurysm rebleeds, there is a significant risk that the person will die or be left with a major disability. Therefore, after an aneurysm ruptures, there is rarely a place for observation alone as a treatment option. Even elderly patients can usually tolerate either open surgery or coiling, and with the very high risk of potentially fatal rebleeding, most patients are candidates for some form of therapy to repair the aneurysm. Rare exceptions may include patients with a terminal or chronic, debilitating illness who may prefer to accept the risk of rebleeding rather than undergo a surgical procedure.

Based on these facts, the real question for most patients who've suffered aneurysm rupture is not whether to treat the aneurysm but how (clipping vs. coiling). There are no strict guidelines in terms of deciding which treatment option is better for a given case. The answer will depend heavily on the experience levels of the neurosurgeon and the interventional neuroradiologist involved in the case.

As a general rule, the patient is best served if they are treated in a hospital that has both an experienced person who does aneurysm surgery (a vascular neurosurgeon) as well as an experienced person who coils aneurysms (either a neurosurgeon or an interventional neuroradiologist). Furthermore, the patient is best served in a place where the two collaborate as a team rather than function in a competitive manner. In the author's practice, every aneurysm patient that comes to the hospital is evaluated by both the author (a vascular neurosurgeon) and an interventional neuroradiologist. Together, a decision regarding the optimal treatment for the aneurysm can be decided upon and then relayed to the patient and family. As a general rule, elderly patients and those patients who are in poor condition because of a severe hemorrhage will often do well with coiling. This avoids putting the patient through an open surgical procedure which is somewhat more stressful to the system of an elderly or very ill patient. Open surgery requires lifting up the brain to reach the aneurysm, and after a severe hemorrhage, the brain may be very swollen and may not tolerate the surgery well.

Also as a rule, young patients and those in good condition after a mild or moderate hemorrhage tend to do well after surgical clipping of the aneurysm. The advantage of surgery as discussed already is its proven track record in comparison with coiling. The author typically makes a decision in each case as to whether he can successfully clip the aneurysm without undue risk to the patient. If the answer is yes, then surgery is typically preferred because the risk of recurrence is so much lower with open surgery than with coiling. If the answer is no, then it may be best to accept the long-term risk of a late recurrence rather than go ahead with a risky surgery that is likely to result in a serious injury to the patient (who may not be very thankful that the aneurysm is gone for good after surgery if he or she is left with a permanent paralysis or other major disability).

Again, this type of decision will depend heavily on the experience of the surgeon. An inexperienced surgeon who rarely operates on aneurysms may have very high complication rates from surgery and should probably not be involved in treatment decision making because he/she is not in a position to properly assess the risks of surgery in the hands of a more experienced surgeon. Ideally, the inexperienced surgeon should refer the aneurysm patient to a vascular neurosurgeon rather than referring the patient for coiling or simply going ahead with an ill-advised surgery.

In addition, it should be noted that certain aneurysm locations are usually better treated with open surgery. Aneurysms located on the middle cerebral artery are a good example of this. These aneurysms seem to carry a high risk of stroke when treated with coiling. Aneurysms located on the basilar artery are particularly dangerous with surgery and are much riskier than aneurysms at other locations. Only highly experienced surgeons and those with special training should operate on aneurysms in this location. Although these aneurysms are often easy to coil, they also have a high tendency to regrow after coiling; therefore, these aneurysms represent a particular challenge and deserve to be managed by neurosurgeons and neuroradiologists with special expertise.

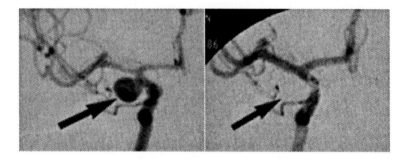

Figures 9 A&B. These are actual angiogram images obtained in a patient who presented with the sudden onset of severe headache associated with loss of consciousness. Figure 9A shows a large, ruptured aneurysm (arrow) on the internal carotid artery. In Figure 9B, the aneurysm is no longer seen after surgical clipping (arrow inserted in similar location for comparison purposes). Figure 9B is an image from an intraoperative angiogram, an angiogram obtained in the operating room before the skull was closed. Of note, the clip itself is not seen because the angiogram "subtracts" out the metal of the clip to give a better image.

Unruptured Aneurysms

The decision-making process for unruptured aneurysms is even more difficult because observation alone becomes an important consideration. As discussed in Chapter 3, we used to think that unruptured aneurysms bled at a rate of 1–2% per year. Because of this, most patients other than the elderly and infirm, underwent elective, prophylactic repair of unruptured aneurysms to avoid the cumulative risk of future rupture.

The results of a large study of patients with unruptured aneurysms (the International Study on Unruptured Intracranial Aneurysms) now seem to suggest that aneurysms bleed less often than we'd previously thought. The final data will not be available for several more years, but preliminary results suggest that small unruptured aneurysms may bleed at significantly lower rates, possibly as low as 0.05% per year.

This represents a very difficult problem because the likelihood of the aneurysm ever bleeding may be small, but the consequences of bleeding (should it ever occur) are quite severe. In general, elderly patients or those with a short life expectancy who are found to have aneurysms that have never bled and that are not causing symptoms are best treated by observation alone in most cases. Young and middle-aged patients are considered for treatment, but the specific risks and complications of surgery and coiling as well as the likelihood of future rupture should all be discussed openly with the patient in order to reach an appropriate decision. This will depend heavily on the experience of the surgeon or interventional radiologist.

In the setting of unruptured aneurysms, the surgeon's primary responsibility is to honestly assess his/her own capabilities to repair the aneurysm without causing significant disability. It makes little sense (and is ethically wrong) for the surgeon to recommend an operation to clip an aneurysm that has a low risk of ever bleeding in the future if the surgeon knows that he or she will likely cause the patient a significant, lifelong disability. This is where the surgeon's personal experience and surgical results become important in the decision making process. Again, surgeons with little experience and no special training in the management of aneurysms should consider referring these patients to vascular neurosurgeons who have greater expertise with these specific problems.

Unruptured Symptomatic Aneurysms

It should be noted that the above discussion on unruptured aneurysms pertains specifically to those aneurysms that have never bled and that are discovered incidentally i.e. that are picked up by accident and not because they're causing any symptoms.

As mentioned in Chapter 2, rarely, aneurysms will be discovered because they cause symptoms other than bleeding. Aneurysms, particularly large and giant ones, may put pressure on the brain or the nerves coming out of the brain and cause either headache, seizure, or loss of normal brain function (weakness, numbness, visual loss, double vision, etc.) much like a tumor that's pressing on the brain. Occasionally, an aneurysm may develop some clot inside and the clot can travel out of the aneurysm and block off a brain artery causing a stroke. In these cases, treatment with either surgery or coiling is usually the rule with the specific recommendations being dictated by the individual situation.

The sudden onset of symptoms from an aneurysm (e.g. double vision) may signify the rapid expansion of an aneurysm. This constitutes an urgent situation and may herald a potential rupture if the aneurysm is left untreated. The person should be admitted to the hospital for urgent surgery or coiling of the aneurysm.

Large and giant aneurysms are often better treated with open surgery rather than coiling because it may be hard to insert coils into the aneurysm without having the coils come back out into the main artery upon which the aneurysm is located. In addition, these aneurysms may require special surgical techniques (as described in Chapter 3) such as bypass and trapping to treat the aneurysm.

Activity Restrictions

If someone has an unruptured aneurysm and a decision is made not to treat it, what restrictions should be placed on the individual to decrease the risk of future rupture? The answer will depend on the neurosurgeon asked, but there is a fair bit of evidence to suggest that no real restrictions should be imposed on these patients. Of all aneurysms that bleed, one-third do so during strenuous activity, one-third at rest, and one-third during sleep. In fact, studies have shown severe blood pressure fluctuations during REM sleep that are probably as great as any that occur during routine physical activity.

Although it may make some sense to limit activities that include severe straining such as weight-lifting, it remains unclear whether this will really make a difference in the risk of rupture in this situation. If the aneurysm were so thin and tenuous that routine exercise would result in bleeding, it will probably rupture no matter what restrictions are placed on the patient. The patient should consult with their neurosurgeon to address this topic specifically in each individual case.

CHAPTER 6

Additional Commonly Asked Questions

About Aneurysms

What is a stroke and how is it different from aneurysm rupture?

A stroke is a general term that refers to a loss of brain function because something goes wrong inside an artery supplying blood flow to the brain. Most commonly, this is an embolism that may come from the heart or from the carotid arteries in the neck and travels up and blocks a small artery in the brain. This stops the blood flow to a particular part of the brain and causes a "stroke". In loose terms, aneurysm rupture is a form of a stroke. In reality, SAH or aneurysm rupture refers specifically to the situation in which a "blister" on an artery at the base of the brain actually ruptures. There are many similarities between stroke and SAH, but technically they refer to different problems.

How long has the aneurysm been there?

It is impossible to know how long most aneurysms have been present prior to bleeding. Some may have been there for years, some for shorter periods of time.

Is the aneurysm still bleeding now?

No! The aneurysm typically bleeds for just a few seconds and then stops as a clot forms at the site of rupture.

Could anything have been done sooner to prevent the aneurysm from bleeding?

Possibly. If the aneurysm had been found before bleeding, a surgery or coiling procedure might have prevented the bleeding. Nevertheless, most aneurysms aren't discovered until they bleed.

Will the patient ever be the same again?

This is very individualized based on the patient and the severity of hemorrhage. It can take more than a year to fully recover from a severe hemorrhage, and some subtle changes may persist even in those who make an otherwise excellent recovery after aneurysm rupture.

Are we at the right hospital to have this taken care of?

This is a very difficult question and depends mostly on the hospital and the surgeon and the number of patients with aneurysms he/she typically cares for on an annual basis. In general, the more patients the surgeon has treated, and the higher the volume of aneurysm patients seen at that hospital, the more likely they are to be able to properly manage this problem. There are no absolute guidelines regarding numbers or experience, but there are neurosurgeons who specialize in vascular neurosurgery and aneurysms. These surgeons treat a large number of patients with aneurysms and are probably best qualified to manage this problem. In one recent article in the Journal of the American Medical Association, centers that cared for fewer than 30 aneurysm patients per year had twice as many deaths as those centers that cared for more than 30 patients per year.

Also, ideally, the case should be reviewed by a neurosurgeon highly skilled in open surgery and a neurosurgeon or neuroradiologist experienced with aneurysm coiling. By working as a team, the two can recommend the ideal treatment for each patient. In some hospitals, the neurosurgeon and neuroradiologist may function in a "competitive" manner. This is suboptimal because the two won't work together to recommend the best treatment; rather, each will tend to recommend their technique (open surgery vs. coiling) as best.

What questions should we ask the surgeon to know if he/she is qualified to handle this problem?

This is a related and important question. It would be reasonable to ask the surgeon whether they specialize in vascular neurosurgery. If they don't, is there another person in town who does? Do they have any special training such as a fellowship in aneurysm surgery? A fellowship means the surgeon spent an additional period of time (usually a year) studying a specific area of neurosurgery. Also, how many aneurysms per year do they operate upon? Fewer than 10–20 is probably too few. Do they collaborate with a neurosurgeon or neuroradiologist who does coiling? Will they review the films together, and can you meet with that person to discuss your case? Finally, it may be worthwhile to ask to speak with their three most recent patients who've had aneurysm surgery. If they have to go back a year to find three names, you're probably at the wrong place.

Most cities have at least one neurosurgeon who has special training in aneurysm surgery. Especially if the aneurysm is unruptured and there's no rush to get it treated, it may be worthwhile to find this person, at least to get his/her opinion.

Are aneurysms hereditary? Should family members be checked?

Aneurysms can be hereditary and can run in families. Most often, this is well known to the family members who are fully aware that a number of people within the family have had ruptured aneurysms. We typically recommend screening for family members if there are two first degree relatives in the family with known aneurysms. Screening can usually be done non-invasively with MRI/MRA (see glossary for details).

Will the aneurysm ever come back?

If an aneurysm is successfully clipped with surgery and an angiogram during or after surgery shows that it is gone, the likelihood of it ever coming back is extremely small (probably less than 1%). In this instance, the patient is considered cured and never needs special follow-up testing. If there is residual aneurysm on the angiogram, a decision is made by the surgeon whether to recommend another operation, coiling of the residual, or observation with follow-up.

If a patient has their aneurysm coiled, then the chance of recurrence is much higher, and a detailed discussion is located in chapters 3 and 5. Careful follow-up with angiography is necessary after coiling because the aneurysm can regrow.

Which treatment is best, surgery or coiling?

This is a very complex question that is discussed in detail in chapters 3 and 5.

My doctor tells me I have an infundibulum. What is that? Is it an aneurysm?

An infundibulum is not a true aneurysm. Rather, an infundibulum is a dilation of the origin of a small artery as it arises from a larger artery at the base of the brain. The most common location is the origin of the posterior communicating artery coming directly off the main carotid artery just after it enters the skull. The small artery seems to start out a bit "swollen" before narrowing back down to normal size.

To the best of our knowledge, an infundibulum is a safe variant of normal anatomy. They almost never bleed (possibly never at all), and are not considered dangerous. No treatment is recommended for an infundibulum.

Are there any medicines or vitamins I can take to make the aneurysm go away?

Not that we know of. An aneurysm is a thinned-out part of the wall of an artery, and once it forms, we don't have any medicine that can make it regress or make the wall of the artery tough again.

PART II

VASCULAR MALFORMATIONS OF THE BRAIN

CHAPTER 7

Vascular Malformations –Basic Definitions

What is a vascular malformation of the brain?

Up to this point, we have focused our discussion on brain aneurysms. As you should know by now, a brain aneurysm is a focal area of dilatation involving the wall of an artery at the base of the brain. The primary abnormality appears to be a specific area of weakness in the wall of the artery; this point of weakness allows the wall to gradually dilate over time resulting in the development of an aneurysm. It should be noted, however, that the actual pattern of development of the arteries and veins is basically normal in these patients. This is not true in the patient with a vascular malformation.

To understand the concept of a vascular malformation, we need to return to a basic review of how blood flows from the heart to the brain and then back to the heart. Remember the story about Mr. Johnson and his new house. There were pipes that carried fresh water from the water plant, and then there were complimentary pipes that carried the dirty water back to the plant. Extending this analogy to the human body, you may recall that the water plant represents the heart which pumps the blood to the brain. The arteries bring the blood flow up to the brain and then branch repeatedly into progressively smaller arteries. The smallest arteries are also known as arterioles. These arterioles branch even more, emptying their blood flow into thin-walled channels known as capillaries. The walls of capillaries are so thin that they allow the oxygen and the nutrients of the blood to be transferred to the surrounding brain tissue.

After the blood in the capillaries gives off its nutrients, it empties into tiny veins also known as venules. Multiple venules come together to form small veins, and small veins join together to form progressively larger veins. Eventually, the large veins drain out of the skull to become the jugular veins in the neck carrying blood flow back toward the heart.

This is the normal pattern of development for the blood vessels, the arteries, veins, and capillaries, of the brain. The blood flows to the brain inside the large arteries under high pressure. As the arteries branch into smaller arteries and then arterioles, the pressure gradually becomes lower. At the level of the capillaries, the pressure is even lower, and this helps allow the brain to transfer the nutrients and oxygen from the bloodstream. The pressure in the veins is even lower than in the capillaries.

A vascular malformation of the brain represents a maldevelopment of either the arteries, veins, or capillaries in a specific part of the brain. This chapter provides a basic overview of the different types of vascular malformations of the brain. Each will be discussed further in the following chapters. The malformations that cause the most trouble from a medical perspective, arteriovenous malformations and cavernous malformations, will be discussed in the most detail.

What are the Different Types of Vascular Malformations?

There are four basic types of vascular malformations that occur in the brain: 1. arteriovenous malformations (AVMs), 2. cavernous malformations (also known as cavernous angiomas or cavernomas), 3. capillary telangiectasias, and 4. venous angiomas (also known as developmental venous anomalies or DVAs).

The different types of vascular malformations have differing characteristic appearances to the naked eye and on radiologic testing. They behave differently, and their treatment needs to be addressed on an individualized basis. Capilllary telangiectasias and venous angiomas almost never cause symptoms. They are usually discovered by accident either at the time of autopsy or by MRI scan. Cavernous malformations and AVMs may cause seizures or bleeding within the brain, and AVMs in particular are potentially quite dangerous.

AVMs

Arteriovenous malformations or AVMs are abnormal collections of arteries and veins typically located within the substance of the brain itself. They are described in great detail in Chapters 8 & 9. AVMs appear to be associated with a lack of or an inappropriate development of the capillaries that normally connect the arteries to the veins within the brain. When the capillaries fail to form normally, the blood which is flowing under high pressure in the arteries, empties directly into the veins without passing through the smaller caliber capillary channels. Because the veins are normally thin-walled compared to the arteries, they are not designed to carry high pressure blood flow the way that arteries do.

In AVMs, the blood flows into the veins under abnormally high pressure, and therefore, the blood vessel walls may weaken over time and eventually rupture. This can cause bleeding which results in the development of a blood clot inside the brain. Such a blood clot is also known as an intracerebral hemorrhage. "Intra" means in, "cerebral" means brain, and "hemorrhage" means bleeding. If the deepest part of the AVM extends to the fluid-filled cavities (ventricles) deep within the brain, it can cause bleeding into the ventricles or an "intraventricular hemorrhage". In addition, AVMs can cause irritation of the surrounding brain, resulting in seizures or the gradual loss of normal brain function. Again, this will be discussed in detail in the following chapters.

Cavernous malformations

Cavernous malformations are small clusters of abnormal, thin-walled blood vessels that can occur anywhere within the substance of the brain. When removed at the time of surgery or autopsy, the cavernous malformation resembles a small cluster of darkly colored grapes or a mulberry. Cavernous malformations have a tendency to bleed repeatedly into themselves. These repeated "microhemorrhages" are rarely life-threatening because the bleeding is often contained within the confines of the lesion. The malformations tend to enlarge gradually over time, growing a bit each time they bleed into themselves.

Cavernous malformations come to medical attention because of these repeated hemorrhages. The bleeding can cause seizures or headaches or loss of neurological function. Interestingly, a relatively high proportion of individuals with cavernous malformations have multiple malformations, and there is a strong predilection for this particular type of vascular malformation to run in families.

Cavernous malformations may be visible on CT scan, but they are seen most easily on MRI scanning. Interestingly, because the flow of blood within cavernous malformations is extremely sluggish, these lesions only rarely show up on routine angiograms. This is an important point and will be discussed in detail below. Cavernous malformations are found next to venous angiomas in a large percentage of cases, and this will also be discussed further.

Venous angiomas—Developmental venous anomalies

A venous angioma is also known as a developmental venous anomaly because the term "angioma" implies a "growth" which does not properly describe this type of malformation. In fact, a venous angioma is really nothing more than a group of veins that drain a normal portion of the brain but that have formed in a funny, aberrant pattern. To the best of our knowledge, a venous angioma is a small group of veins that develops in an unusual pattern and that is present from the time of birth. The venous channels of a venous angioma are intrinsically normal. They have normal walls and are of normal size; they simply come together in a funny pattern.

Normally, the capillaries empty their blood into the tiny veins known as venules. Venules join together with other venules to form small veins. The small veins join together to form larger and then larger veins, eventually forming large veins on the surface of the brain which drain out of the skull. The pattern of development is different in a venous angioma. In the patient with a venous angioma, multiple small veins drain directly into a single large vein that itself runs through the substance of the brain to reach the surface. This characteristic pattern is easily recognized on MRI scanning or with an angiogram. Because the multiple small veins draining into the angioma form a radial or circular pattern, the appearance of the venous angioma has traditionally been described as a spoke-and-wheel pattern or a "caput medusa" after the head of the Greek figure with snakes in her hair.

The patient with a venous angioma has normally formed arteries and capillaries, with normal blood flowing to the brain. The blood then empties from the capillaries into the veins, but in the region of the venous angioma, the blood flows through the abnormal pattern of small veins that make up the venous angioma. It is important to recognize that the venous angioma provides the only drainage of blood flow for its particular area of the brain. Removing a venous angioma removes this drainage pathway and can cause a dangerous buildup of back-pressure within the arteries and capillaries, potentially causing bleeding into the brain itself. Because venous angiomas almost never cause symptoms, and because their removal is potentially hazardous, venous angiomas should not be removed surgically. This will be discussed in detail in Chapter 11. The frequent association between cavernous malformations and venous angiomas has been mentioned already and will also be discussed further.

Capillary telangiectasias

Capillary telangiectasias are tiny collections of capillaries that form inappropriately deep within the substance of the brain. They often develop in a part of the brainstem known as the pons. They are so small that it is almost impossible to see them on CT scanning, and even a high quality MRI scan will miss most capillary telangiectasias. Capillary telangiectasias rarely, if ever, cause symptoms. Because they almost never cause symptoms and because it is almost impossible to identify them (other than when they are found by accident at the time of an autopsy), capillary telangiectasias are probably the least important of the vascular malformations from a medical perspective. They will be discussed in limited detail in Chapter 11.

How dangerous are vascular malformations of the brain?

"Natural history" is a medical term for the way in which a disease process will behave if left untreated. Some illnesses or lesions have "benign" natural histories, in other words they are not very dangerous even without any treatment. Certainly, if the natural history is quite benign and the treatment options carry a significant risk, it may be most reasonable to leave things alone. Other lesions will have a more rapidly progressive or "malignant" natural history. In these cases, aggressive intervention to attempt to alter the disease's natural history is appropriate. The worse the natural history of a disease, the more risk a patient and physician may be willing to accept in its treatment.

For example, we've already spent a fair bit of time discussing the natural history of brain aneurysms. Although there is still quite a bit that we don't know, it is well established that the natural history of a ruptured brain aneurysm is quite poor. The risk of rebleeding is very high; the consequences of this rebleeding are severe. Therefore, aggressive treatment with surgery or coiling is warranted, even though these procedures each carry a small, but definite risk of stroke or death.

Therefore, whenever a physician evaluates the treatment options for a particular disorder, he or she must take into account the natural history of the disease. The different vascular malformations mentioned above have differing natural histories. Capillary telangiectasias and venous angiomas rarely, if ever, cause symptoms. They are not thought to pose a danger to the patient. On the other hand, cavernous malformations can cause seizures or small hemorrhages. Our best data suggest they bleed at a rate of approximately 0.5–2% per year. That means that each year, a person with a cavernous malformation has a risk somewhere between 1 in 200 and 1 in 50 of suffering a hemorrhage.

It must be remembered, however, that when a cavernous malformation bleeds, the consequences are rarely serious. In comparison, bleeding from a cavernous malformation is typically much less significant than when an aneurysm bleeds. This will be reviewed in detail in Chapter 10. Although aneurysm rupture carries a 50% chance of death and a major risk of permanent disability in survivors, bleeding from a cavernous malformation results in death or major permanent disability in only a small percentage of individuals, probably less than 5%, and maybe less than 1% of cases. Therefore, the risk of serious injury from bleeding from a cavernous malformation is low.

In addition, it appears that not all cavernous malformations will behave in similar fashion. Mr. Jones may have a cavernous malformation located in the frontal lobe that bleeds five times in one year, while Mr. Smith has a cavernous malformation in the frontal lobe that bleeds once and then remains silent for 5 years. Clearly, the risk of future rebleeding is very different for these individuals, although it might have been difficult for us to predict in advance that Mr. Jones' cavernous malformation would behave so differently than Mr. Smith's. This is something we don't understand.

At times, particularly when a cavernous malformation is located in an area that makes surgery dangerous, it may be reasonable to follow things over time to get a sense for how that particular malformation will behave. If there are multiple hemorrhages over a short period of time as in Mr. Jones' case, treatment may be indicated. Alternatively, if the lesion remains quiescent as in Mr. Smith's case, we might well decide to leave it alone. Like many decisions regarding the treatment of brain lesions, things are rarely as simple as they might seem.

Finally, AVMs represent the most potentially dangerous type of vascular malformations of the brain. AVMs can cause seizures, bleeding, or loss of brain function. Although bleeding from an AVM tends to have less severe consequences than that from an aneurysm, it is typically much worse than that from a cavernous malformation. Our best data indicate that AVMs bleed at a rate between 1% and 3% per year. Each time an AVM bleeds, there is a 10% risk of death and a 30% risk of permanent disability (less severe than with an aneurysm, but still quite serious). Most people with bleeding from an AVM develop a severe headache and some neurologic dysfunction (weakness, numbness, visual disturbance, speech difficulty) which requires a hospital stay followed by some rehabilitation. This usually resolves over time. The management of AVMs is a very complex subject and will be reviewed in detail in Chapter 9.

What are the Treatment Options for Vascular Malformations?

There are four major treatment options for vascular malformations of the brain. These may be used independently or in combination with one another. As mentioned already, the first question is whether any treatment at all is appropriate. The first major option in the management of a vascular malformation (as we encountered with an aneurysm) is observation alone. This means the malformation is left untreated and possibly followed with additional MRI scanning over time. The second option is surgical removal of the malformation. This is performed by an open operation in which the malformed blood vessels are cauterized and then removed from the brain.

The third treatment option is radiation. As you may know, radiation can injure and even block off blood vessels within the human body. If administered properly, a highly focused dose of high energy radiation has the ability to cause the gradual obliteration of certain vascular malformations, particularly AVMs. This is a complex technique that will be reviewed in detail along with the management options for AVMs of the brain.

The final option is known as embolization. Like aneurysm coiling, this technique is performed by a neurosurgeon or neuroradiologist who performs an angiogram and passes the catheter all the way up into the artery that supplies blood flow to the malformation. At this point, the specific artery feeding the malformation can be "embolized" or blocked off with an artificial substance such as glue or metal coils. This will decrease the blood flow to the malformation. In rare cases, this may be curative. More commonly, the flow is decreased but not completely shut off. Surgery or radiosurgery may then be used to treat the remaining malformation.

Where are Vascular Malformations Located?

You may recall that aneurysms are located underneath the brain on the large arteries carrying blood flow to the brain. In contrast, vascular malformations are located within the brain itself. They can develop anywhere that arteries, veins, and capillaries are located, therefore, they can be found in every part of the brain. Of note, capillary telangiectasias seem to have a predilection for deep parts of the brain including the brainstem, and venous angiomas tend to be found deep within the brain, often close to the fluid cavities in the center of the brain, the ventricles. AVMs often extend from the surface of the brain down toward its center in a cone-shaped fashion, and this will be expanded upon below. Finally, cavernous malformations may be located anywhere in the brain in both superficial and deep locations.

How Common are Vascular Malformations?

Vascular malformations are relatively common. The exact incidence of these lesions is not certain, because many individuals have them but never know it. In particular, capillary telangiectasias are very difficult to find other than by autopsy, so their exact incidence can only be determined using autopsy studies.

In general, it appears that AVMs of the brain are about one-tenth as common as aneurysms. If one adds up all patients with AVMS, cavernous malformations, venous angiomas, and capillary telangiectasias, between 0.5% and 5% of individuals probably have a vascular malformation of the brain.

Why do Vascular Malformations Form?

As discussed already, we believe that aneurysms of the brain develop at sites where an inherent point of weakness within the wall of an artery gradually dilates over time to form an aneurysm. The person may be born with a predisposition for the development of the aneurysm but not with the aneurysm itself.

In contrast, we believe that vascular malformations are true abnormalities in the pattern of development of the blood vessels of the brain. This will be discussed in greater detail in association with each particular malformation. Whereas aneurysms are almost never found in infants and children, it is common for vascular malformations to be seen early in life, further suggesting that they are congenital abnormalities i.e. that people are born with them. Certain diseases such as Osler-Weber-Rendu or Hereditary Hemorrhagic Telangiectasia result in the development of multiple AVMs both in the brain and also in other parts of the body such as the lungs and the skin. Again, this represents further evidence that AVMs are basically congenital lesions.

Using our old analogy, if Mr. Johnson had messed up while he was installing the pipes for his water, accidentally connecting up the pipes incorrectly so that the pattern of water flow no longer proceeded properly from the inflow pipes to the faucets and sinks, and then to the outflow pipes, he would have created a situation akin to a vascular malformation of the brain. Stay tuned for more details on this.

Can one Person Have Multiple Vascular Malformations?

A small percentage of individuals will have more than one vascular malformation. This varies depending on the type of malformation involved. AVMs almost always occur in isolation i.e. without the presence of a venous angioma, capillary telangiectasia, or a cavernous malformation. There have been rare cases of AVMs associated with a venous angioma, and the exact relationship between the two in these instances is uncertain. Capillary telangiectasias typically occur in isolation as well.

On the other hand, cavernous malformations often occur in direct association with a venous angioma. This happens so commonly that it is likely that there is a direct relationship between the two lesions. Of note, venous angiomas are often found alone, but cavernous malformations are typically found next to a venous angioma. The treatment of patients with multiple vascular malformations, particularly those with cavernous malformations and venous angiomas (by far the most common combination) is discussed in the Chapter 10.

Can one Person Have an Aneurysm and a Vascular Malformation?

Yes. Approximately 10% of people with an AVM also have an aneurysm. In the majority of cases, the aneurysms are located on an artery that continues on to deliver blood flow to the AVM. As will be explained in the next chapter, a tremendous and very abnormal amount of blood often flows through an AVM of the brain. The arteries of the brain are only designed to handle a certain amount of blood flow. The increased flow associated with an AVM can "overload" the wall of the artery that must carry that blood flow, and eventually, an aneurysm can form. Think back to Mr. Johnson's house. If he kept all his faucets running all the time at full water power, the area of weakness in the rubber tubing would have started to give out that much sooner. In the same way, the increased flow associated with an AVM probably causes an inherent point of weakness to show up as an area of dilation, an aneurysm. Of note, the aneurysms found with AVMs are often fusiform in nature (see chapter 1, figure 2) because the entire wall of the artery (not just a focal point) can dilate under the increased flow demands of the AVM.

Occasionally, aneurysms are found on blood vessels remote from the AVM. The association of the aneurysm and AVM in these cases is uncertain. It may be that these individuals have multiple "unrelated" abnormalities due to a genetic defect that affects the structure of the arteries of the brain. Finally, aneurysms may also be found on the abnormal arteries and veins deep within an AVM. In these cases, the aneurysms are probably just dilated portions of grossly abnormal blood vessels that never formed normally in the first place. The treatment of aneurysms related to AVMs will be discussed in Chapter 9.

There is no known association between aneurysms and vascular malformations other than AVMs. Because aneurysms are relatively common, and cavernous malformations, venous angiomas, and capillary telangiectasias are as well, the rare individual will be found to have an aneurysm and also one of these lesions. In these cases, it seems that the lesions coexist by chance rather than because of a direct association between the two.

CHAPTER 8

Arteriovenous Malformations (AVMs) of the Brain

What is an AVM?

AVM is short for artery-vein malformation or arteriovenous malformation. An AVM is one of the specific types of vascular malformations that may be found in the brain. To properly understand AVMs, we must again return to the basic structure of the arteries and veins of the brain, as we did in the preceding chapter.

When Mr. Johnson constructed his house, he installed tubing to carry fresh water from the water plant to his house and also complimentary tubing to carry the dirty water back to the plant. In the human body, the heart acts as the central "water plant" pumping enriched blood (which carries oxygen and other nutrients) to all parts of the body including the brain. The (carotid and vertebral) arteries are thick-walled channels that bring the blood flow to the brain. They branch repeatedly into progressively smaller arteries to reach all parts of the brain. The smallest arteries are also known as arterioles. These arterioles branch even more, emptying their blood flow into extremely thin-walled channels known as capillaries. The walls of the capillaries are so thin that the oxygen and nutrients in the blood inside the capillaries can diffuse or pass through the walls and into the surrounding brain tissue.

After the blood in the capillaries gives off its nutrients, it empties into tiny veins known as venules. Multiple venules come together to form small veins, and small veins join together to form progressively larger veins. Eventually, the large veins drain out of the skull to become the jugular veins in the neck. The jugular veins carry blood flow back to the heart, where it can be "recycled" to be pumped back to the body once again.

This is the normal pattern of development for the blood vessels of the brain. The blood reaches the brain inside the large arteries under very high pressure. Remember, if you cut an artery, you can bleed to death because of the high pressure, while a cut in a vein is rarely dangerous because the pressure in the veins is so much lower. A bit of gentle pressure held over a cut in a vein is all that's needed to stop the bleeding.

As the arteries branch into smaller arteries and then arterioles, the pressure gradually becomes lower. At the level of the capillaries, the pressure is even lower, and the pressure in the veins is even lower than in the capillaries. An AVM is technically a disordered tangle of arteries and veins located in a particular part of the brain. AVMs appear to be associated with a maldevelopment of the capillaries (the vessels that connect the arteries and veins) in that part of the brain. When the capillaries don't form properly, blood flows under high arterial pressure directly from the arteries into the veins (Figure 10). Remember that the thin-walled veins are not designed to carry blood flow under such high pressure. This point will become important when we discuss why AVMs are potentially dangerous lesions.

AVMs can occur anywhere that arteries and veins are found, in other words, they can occur anywhere in the substance of the brain. The "classic" AVM extends from the surface of the brain in cone-shaped fashion down to the center of the brain, ending at the level of the ventricle, the fluid-filled cavity at the center of the brain. Some AVMs don't reach the surface of the brain, others don't reach the ventricle. Some are very small, and others can be quite large (the size of an orange or greater). No two AVMs are identical in shape, size, and location. The defining features of an AVM include its location in the brain, its size, and its blood supply. Understanding the blood supply of an AVM includes a recognition of which arteries carry blood to the AVM and which veins drain blood away from the AVM. These features will determine the surgeons' ability to treat a particular AVM and will be discussed further below.

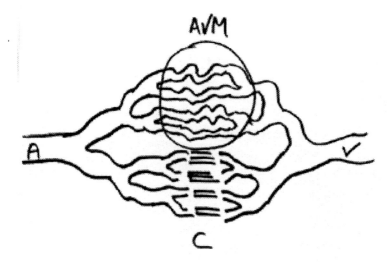

Figure 10. This drawing illustrates a large artery (A) dividing into progressively smaller arteries that normally empty into tiny capillaries (C, at the bottom). The capillaries empty into small veins that join with other small veins to empty into a large vein (V). At the top, an AVM is circled where the arteries are directly connected to the veins without the presence of normal capillary channels. Note how the AVM receives blood flow from the same main artery as the normal arteries below. Also, the normal arteries, capillaries, and veins at the bottom ultimately empty their blood flow into the same vein as the AVM. This will become important below when we discuss how AVMs can "steal" blood flow from nearby normal areas of the brain and how AVMs can cause a buildup of pressure in the vein (V) that also drains the blood flow from normal arteries and veins in the vicinity.

Why Do AVMs Develop?

The truth is we don't fully understand why AVMs form. As already described, we believe that AVMs are, in general, congenital lesions. This means that they form because of a problem with development before birth. It may be that the primary problem is that the capillaries in that part of the brain don't form properly, resulting in an abnormal connection between the arteries and veins in that spot, but this is just a theory.

It is likely that there is some genetic basis for AVM development. There are certain diseases such as Osler-Weber-Rendu or Hereditary-Hemorrhagic-Telangiectasia in which the patient has multiple AVMs in different parts of the body including the brain, the lungs, and the skin. This is a disease that has been associated with an abnormality in a gene on chromosome number 5. We don't know what this particular gene is supposed to do, but it seems that when the gene is not functioning properly, the patient develops AVMs. In the future, if we can identify the reason that AVMs develop, we may be able to prevent them from forming by screening for the genetic defect and then repairing it in utero (in the mother's uterus). For now, we have to treat AVMs that have already fully developed.

How Dangerous are AVMs?

AVMs are potentially very dangerous lesions. Because AVMs are located within the substance of the brain, when an AVM bleeds, the blood escapes into the brain itself causing a blood clot in the brain. Bleeding from an AVM carries a mortality rate of approximately 10%. In other words, about 10% of people die when their AVM bleeds. In addition, roughly 30% of people are left with some permanent disability after an AVM bleeds. These numbers are nowhere near as high as those associated with bleeding from a brain aneurysm, but they still make AVMs potentially dangerous. This will be discussed in detail below.

How Do People Find out They Have an AVM?

Incidental Finding

AVMs may be discovered in a number of different ways. First, they may be identified by accident if a person is having a CT or MRI scan for an unrelated reason. For example, AVMs are occasionally picked up when a person has a CT scan following a motor vehicle accident. In these cases, the AVM is said to be an incidental (accidental) finding.

Headache

AVMs may cause chronic migraine-type headaches prompting a scan that identifies the malformation as the source of the headaches. We don't really understand why AVMs cause headaches. The reason probably relates to the increased blood flow through the AVM.

Some AVMs derive part or all of their blood supply from the dura mater, the tough covering of the brain. The dura is heavily innervated, in other words, the dura has many nerve endings and is very sensitive to pain. The increased blood flow through the blood vessels within the dura may be responsible for the headache in these cases. In patients who have a lot of their blood supply coming from the dura, stopping this part of the blood supply with surgery or embolization (see below) will often reduce significantly the persons' headaches, even if the rest of the AVM is left in place.

Bleeding

AVMs often come to medical attention when they bleed. The risk of an AVM bleeding appears to be somewhere between 1% and 3% per year. Therefore, every year, the person with an AVM has a 1/100 to 3/100 risk that they will have bleeding from their AVM. It should be noted, however, that not all AVMs behave the same way. Some AVMs appear to have a high risk of bleeding and will bleed repeatedly until they are treated. Others are discovered only by accident at the time of autopsy after a person has lived a full and healthy life. We will talk about some possible explanations for this later in the chapter.

Remember that AVMs are located inside the substance of the brain itself. Therefore, bleeding from an AVM results in blood escaping into the brain, causing a blood clot in the brain. This is also called an intracerebral hematoma or intracerebral hemorrhage. "Intra" means in, "cerebral" means brain, and "hematoma" or "hemorrhage" mean bleeding. At times, if the AVM reaches the fluid-filled cavities in the center of the brain, the ventricles, then the AVM can bleed into the ventricles. This is known as an intraventricular hemorrhage. In contrast, remember that aneurysms are usually located in the space around the brain known as the sub-arachnoid space. Therefore, when an aneurysm bleeds, the blood escapes into this space, filling the spinal fluid with blood. Aneurysms occasionally cause bleeding directly into the brain the way that AVMs do.

In the first few chapters of the book, we reviewed in detail the consequences of aneurysm rupture. You may recall that this is a very dangerous event, resulting in death and permanent disability in well over half of the people who suffer aneurysm rupture. Bleeding from an AVM is different. Each time an AVM bleeds, the risk of death is only approximately 10%. Although more than 50% of people develop a new neurologic deficit (weakness, numbness, vision loss, speech or comprehension difficulty, etc.) at the time of the bleeding, only 30% are left with permanent disability, the majority clearing up with time and rehabilitation. Therefore, bleeding from an AVM can be very serious and can even be life-threatening, but bleeding from an AVM is not as dangerous as bleeding from an aneurysm.

Another important distinguishing feature between aneurysm and AVM bleeding is how the two lesions behave after they bleed. Remember that once an aneurysm bleeds, the risk of rebleeding is extremely high, approaching 40% by 6 months after the initial bleeding. Therefore, after an aneurysm bleeds, treatment of the aneurysm should be performed as soon as possible to prevent it from bleeding again. In contrast, after an AVM bleeds, the risk of the AVM bleeding again is only slightly increased. Therefore, most neurosurgeons will wait four to eight weeks after the bleeding before treating the AVM. This allows the blood clot caused by the AVM to break down and start to be reabsorbed by the body. It also allows the brain to "settle down", so that surgery can be performed under the very best of circumstances. These points will be discussed below in the section on AVM treatment.

It should be noted that if the risk of rebleeding from ruptured aneurysms weren't so high, we would do the same thing with aneurysms, because it would be easier on the patient (and the surgeon) to wait and treat the aneurysm weeks after the bleeding, once any brain swelling has subsided. The problem is if we waited that long, a significant number of people would rebleed and die during the waiting period. .

Neurological Deficit

Occasionally, an AVM can cause symptoms by gradually producing loss of neurological function. The specific symptoms will depend on the exact location of the AVM. If the malformation is located in the occipital lobe (which normally controls vision), then the AVM may cause progressive loss of vision. If the AVM is located in the back part of the left frontal lobe in the area of the brain that controls movement of the right side of the body, then the AVM may cause gradually increasing weakness of the right side of the body.

The exact mechanism by which an AVM can cause gradual loss of brain function is not completely understood. There are two possible mechanisms by which this may occur. The first is known as "vascular steal", the second is "venous hypertension". These are relatively complicated concepts.

Simply put, vascular steal means that the AVM is stealing blood supply from the surrounding brain tissue. Imagine that the blood is flowing in the large arteries at the base of the brain. The arteries branch repeatedly, distributing the blood flow to all parts of the brain. But when an AVM is present in one part of the brain, the large arteries bringing blood supply to the AVM never branch properly. Instead they empty their blood flow straight into the veins. A tremendous amount of blood flows through the AVM and the AVM acts as a "shunt", sucking up a large amount of flow that was meant to supply a whole section of brain surrounding the AVM. This means that the AVM can "steal" blood flow from the brain around it. When this brain doesn't get enough flow, it may not be able to function properly, resulting in loss of neurologic function. In addition, this surrounding brain may become irritable, and this can produce seizures (see below).

"Venous hypertension" means increased pressure within the veins. We already know that AVMs cause blood to reach the veins under higher than normal pressure. Imagine two areas of the brain that receive blood flow from the same set of arteries and drain into the same set of veins (see above, Figure 10). Now imagine that one of those two areas contains an AVM. The AVM passes tremendous blood flow from the arteries directly into the veins. The blood flowing into the normal neighboring brain still has to flow out through the same set of veins, but the pressure within these veins is much higher than normal. This means that the blood may not be able to empty from the normal nearby brain as it should, and this blood can "back up" under some pressure in the normal part of the brain. When the blood can't empty properly in this fashion, the brain may not be able to function normally, and this could possibly cause a neurologic dysfunction.

Seizure

As discussed in a number of other sections in the book, a seizure results from abnormal electrical activity in the brain. The electrical activity typically starts in one particular area of the brain, and if strong enough, it can spread to neighboring parts of the brain. Seizures can range from mild episodes during which the patient stares off into space and loses a few seconds to full blown epileptic fits with the person falling to the ground, losing consciousness, and shaking violently. Many seizures occur while the person is asleep. The person awakens the next morning with sore muscles, and they've often bitten their tongue. The person sleeping next to them may recall a lot of shaking at some time during the night, but may not have realized at the time that it was a seizure.

In any case, AVMs often result in seizures. A CT scan or MRI will then demonstrate the AVM as the cause of the seizures. AVMs may cause seizures in a number of ways. If the AVM bleeds, the sudden increased pressure within the brain from the blood clot can cause irritation of the brain and result in seizures. After an AVM has bled, the residual blood products left behind after the blood clot has been reabsorbed by the body may result in persistent irritation of the brain and predispose to seizures.

Finally, AVMs may cause seizures in the same way they can cause neurologic deficit as described above. "Vascular steal" can result in an inadequate amount of blood flow reaching the areas of the brain surrounding the AVM. Also, "venous hypertension" can cause a build-up of pressure in the veins draining the normal brain surrounding the AVM. Either of these can result in irritation of the surrounding brain and cause seizures.

What Happens When an AVM Bleeds?

This has been covered to a limited degree in the section above on bleeding from AVMs. When an AVM bleeds, blood escapes from inside the abnormal arteries and veins of the malformation and enters the substance of the brain or the fluid spaces of the ventricles. The bleeding continues for some short period of time until a blood clot forms within the brain. The blood clot naturally acts to slow the bleeding and eventually, the bleeding point seals.

The consequences of this type of bleeding depend on how much bleeding occurs and the location of the bleeding itself. Bleeding from an AVM almost always results in the sudden onset of headache, although the headache may not be as sudden in onset or as severe in intensity as that caused by bleeding from an aneurysm. As you'd probably expect, a large blood clot will be more likely to produce symptoms than a small one. The bleeding can cause a seizure or produce a neurologic deficit (weakness, numbness, speech trouble, visual loss, etc.). This type of bleeding may be confused with a stroke, except most stroke patients don't have much if any headache.

If the AVM is located in the front part of the frontal lobe on the right side, even a large amount of bleeding may not cause much in the way of symptoms other than headache. This is because the front part of the right frontal lobe is a relatively "silent" area of the brain. It does not control important brain function (at least, not that we know of at this point), so injury to this area may not cause any obvious problem. On the other hand, even a small amount of bleeding from an AVM located exactly in the "motor area" (the part of the brain that controls movement on the opposite side of the body) in the back part of the right frontal lobe may be enough to result in a complete paralysis of the left side of the body. This paralysis will usually improve over time. Nevertheless, it is important to recognize that the location of an AVM is important in terms of understanding the effects of any bleeding from that AVM and also in terms of assessing the safety of treating the AVM.

The bleeding will usually cause a headache severe enough that the person will want to see a doctor even if there are no other symptoms. Obviously, if there is a seizure or a new disability or if the bleeding results in a loss of consciousness, the person will be brought to a hospital. CT scanning in these cases will reveal the diagnosis of a brain hemorrhage and may suggest the presence of an AVM.

Finally, you may recall from the section on aneurysms, that bleeding into the fluid around the brain can result in the fluid building up abnormally, a condition known as hydrocephalus. This build-up can be life-threatening and may require drainage of the fluid using a small catheter passed through a tiny hole in the skull, through the brain, and into the fluid-filled spaces in the center of the brain. Because AVMs bleed into the ventricles relatively often, bleeding from an AVM can result in the rapid development of hydrocephalus. As with an aneurysm, this hydrocephalus may result in coma and may be life-threatening. In these cases treatment with a ventricular drain or ventriculostomy may be a life-saving maneuver and may need to be performed on an emergency basis.

What Radiology Tests are Used to Diagnose an AVM?

The same tests that are useful in evaluating brain aneurysms (see Chapter 2) are important in the diagnosis of AVMs. Remember that CT is a quick (less than 5 minute), non-invasive test in which the patient lies with his/her head in a large donut. CT provides an excellent quality picture of the brain itself. It is the best test for showing the presence of fresh bleeding. Because it is so quick and easy, and because it is available in almost every hospital, CT is usually the first test performed when bleeding in the brain from any source is suspected. After an AVM has bled, a CT scan will typically show the blood and may give a hint to the presence of the AVM itself. If an AVM has not bled, a CT scan may suggest that there is an AVM within the brain or may simply show a subtle area of abnormality of uncertain significance. In these cases, the next step is usually an MRI.

MRI is a more sophisticated test that takes longer (up to an hour), requires the patient to lie in a long narrow tube (although newer, more "open" MRI scanners are becoming more available), and gives a more detailed picture of the brain. CT uses x-rays to generate the images, while MRI uses magnetic fields without any radiation to provide pictures of the brain. MRI usually does an excellent job of showing the tangled and abnormally enlarged blood vessels of an AVM within the brain. MRI will also show the presence of a blood clot if the AVM has bled recently.

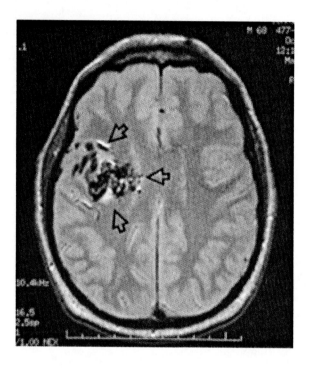

Figure 11. This MR image of the brain demonstrates the typical appearance of a brain AVM. Open arrows have been added to delineate the dark, tortuous blood vessels that make up the malformation. Note how clearly the MRI shows the abnormal blood vessels against the background of the normal brain.

As is the case with aneurysms, the definitive "gold standard" examination to show the details of an AVM is a cerebral arteriogram. As you may recall, an arteriogram (also known as an angiogram) is a test performed by a neuroradiologist or a neurosurgeon. A catheter is passed up from an artery in the groin, through the aorta, all the way to the carotid and vertebral arteries in the neck which supply blood flow to the brain. Dye is injected into each of these arteries as rapid sequence x-ray pictures are taken of the blood vessels in the brain. The arteries and veins of the brain fill with the dye and therefore show up as dark, curving lines on the x-ray images. Any structural abnormality of the arteries and/or veins, including an aneurysm or an AVM, will show up on the arteriogram

The arteriogram also gives additional important information that allows the neurosurgeon to decide on the best mode of treatment for the AVM. The arteriogram shows how much blood flow is traveling through the AVM and exactly which blood vessels are supplying blood flow to the AVM. It also shows if the blood vessels which supply the AVM "dead-end" in the AVM or whether they send off branches to the AVM and then continue on to supply blood to nearby, normal areas of the brain. The arteriogram will show if there are aneurysms associated with the AVM. Finally, the arteriogram will show which veins are draining blood flow from the AVM and if there are any abnormalities of those veins. Sometimes, the vein draining an AVM will have a stricture (a narrowing) that may increase the risk of the AVM bleeding by causing a back-up of blood flow and pressure inside the AVM. All these features become important when planning treatment for an AVM and will be discussed in the next chapter.

Finally, brief mention should be made of CTA and MRA. As you may recall from Chapter 2, these are abbreviations for CT angiogram and MR angiogram. Both test represent specialized software modifications of CT and MRI that allow for the reconstruction of images of the arteries and veins of the brain. They both provide a "poor man's" arteriogram, giving high-resolution pictures of the blood vessels of the brain, but not matching the quality of information provided by a true arteriogram.

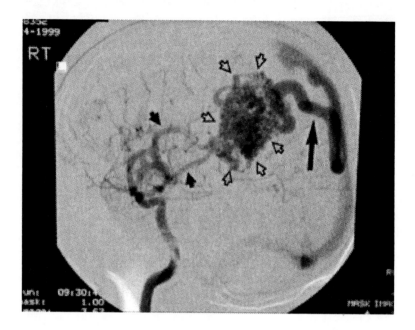

Figure 12. This angiogram reveals a classic AVM. The small dark arrows show the two arteries carrying blood flow to the AVM (the feeding arteries). Open arrows show the compact collection of abnormal blood vessels that make up the AVM itself. Finally the large dark arrow points to the large tortuous vein that drains blood flow away from the AVM.

CHAPTER 9

Treatment Options for Brain AVMs

As in all other sections of this book that discuss treatment options and recommendations for abnormalities of the blood vessels of the brain, this chapter attempts to provide an overview of the basic guidelines which are used by neurosurgeons when they evaluate patients with AVMs of the brain. In no way should this information be regarded as a substitute for consultation with an experienced neurosurgeon because each patient is unique and no two AVMs are exactly alike. A number of options are available when considering treatment for an AVM.

Observation

One of the most important options in the management of the patient with an AVM of the brain is observation alone. Remember that AVMs are congenital lesions, in other words, people are born with them. Today, people are undergoing MRI of the brain for all sorts of reasons, many of which are totally unrelated to the unexpected AVM that turns up by accident on their MRI study. The author has personally been asked to evaluate numerous individuals in their seventies and eighties with the new finding of an asymptomatic AVM, i.e. an AVM that is not producing any symptoms. In these cases, observation is an excellent option. After all, the AVM has probably been there for the person's lifetime, has not caused problems yet, is not likely to cause problems during the patient's expected life span, and treatment carries some risk.

Just as we discussed with aneurysms of the brain, treatment always carries some risk of brain injury, so treatment should only be performed if the risks of treatment are lower than the risks of leaving the AVM alone. Because AVMs of the brain appear to have a more "benign" pattern of behavior than aneurysms, observation alone may be appropriate in a greater percentage of patients with brain AVMs than with aneurysms.

Embolization

Embolization means blocking off an artery from inside the artery itself. In the setting of a brain AVM, embolization is performed by an interventional neuroradiologist or a specially trained neurosurgeon who performs an arteriogram but then passes the catheter all the way up inside the artery as it enters the brain. Once the catheter is positioned inside an artery that supplies blood flow directly to the AVM, past any branches that carry blood flow to the normal brain, material such as glue, metal coils, other particulate matter can be injected directly into the artery. This causes the artery to block off and decreases the blood flow to the AVM.

Most AVMs have multiple arterial feeders, in other words they have multiple arteries bringing blood flow to them. More than one of these arteries can be embolized, depending on the size of the arteries (larger ones are easier to get a catheter into and then embolize) and depending on whether the arteries carrying blood flow to the AVM go on to supply blood flow to normal brain as well. These can't be embolized easily because if they're blocked off, the normal brain they supply would die as well, possibly causing a stroke.

Embolization of a brain AVM can be used for a number of purposes. First, embolization is commonly performed to decrease blood flow to an AVM as a preparatory step before surgery. In this setting, embolization decreases the blood flow in the AVM, and this can make surgery safer by decreasing the blood loss during the operation. Also, preoperative embolization allows for the gradual reduction of blood flow through the AVM, as opposed to sud-denly shutting down the whole AVM at the time of surgery. The concept of gradually decreasing the blood flow through an AVM may be important to prevent a rare complication of surgery known as "normal perfusion pressure breakthrough". This will be discussed below in the section on surgery.

Embolization can be used as a palliative treatment for patients with "inoperable" AVMs. In some cases, surgery would almost certainly result in significant disability because of the size and/or location of an AVM. Some of these patients have severe headaches because of the high blood flow through the AVM, especially when some of the blood flow comes from vessels within the dura, the covering of the brain. Also some of these patients have symptoms of seizures or neurologic dysfunction as discussed in the previous chapter. In these cases, when it is not safe to directly treat the AVM itself, embolization may be used as a palliative measure. This means a non-curative therapy that improves the quality of life for the patient. By decreasing the blood flow through the AVM, some or all of these symptoms may be decreased. Because the AVM is not removed, the blood flow will gradually increase again in most cases, so embolization may have to be repeated every few years in these situations.

Finally, in rare cases, embolization may be able to cure an AVM. This is a complex point. It appears that there are a small number of AVMs which are very simple in nature and may be cured with embolization alone. These AVMs tend to have just one feeding artery and seem to arise as a single large direct con-nection (fistula) between the artery and vein. This type of AVM is also known as an artery-vein fistula or AVF. This can occur in the brain itself or in the dural covering of the brain. At times, these can be cured with just embolization. It should be noted however that the vast majority of AVMs cannot be cured with embolization alone. Most of the time, even after a very aggres-sive attempt to embolize an AVM, the AVM will gradually re-enlarge if it is not removed.

Embolization carries some risk to the patient. First of all, embolization is, by definition, the intentional obstruction of arteries within the brain. As already mentioned, if any artery that is also supplying blood flow to a normal area of the brain is blocked off, a stroke may result. There is also a small chance of injuring and actually rupturing an artery inside the brain with the catheter. Overall, the risk of a serious complication such as stroke or death during embolization of a brain AVM can range from 1% to 8% depending on the complexity of the AVM and the experience of the person performing the procedure.

Microsurgical excision

The surgical removal of a brain AVM is a serious and delicate operation. The procedure is performed, in most cases, with the patient under general anesthesia. An incision is made in the scalp over the area of the skull that overlies the AVM. A window is cut in the skull and the covering of the brain, the dura mater, is then opened. Underneath, the AVM will be visible on the surface of the brain in most cases. The surgeon then works with an operating microscope and uses a cautery device or small metal clips to coagulate or clip off the arteries that are feeding or bringing blood flow to the AVM. After each artery has been cauterized or clipped, it can be divided with scissors.

The surgeon continues in this fashion, working on the surface of the brain, then deeper below the surface, separating the AVM from the surrounding brain tissue. As the surgeon works deeper, he/she continues to cauterize or clip and then divide the feeding arteries. It is important that all the arteries bringing blood flow into the AVM be divided before the veins carrying blood flow away from the AVM are disturbed. If the veins were to be injured early on, the AVM would swell up with blood still entering the AVM from the open arteries, and the AVM would likely burst.

Remember that most AVMs are shaped like cones with the wide base on the surface of the brain, and the point of the cone deep within the brain. The surgeon must continue to work around the outside of the AVM, separating the AVM from the surrounding brain all the way down to the point of the cone. At this point, if the surgery has been done properly, all the arteries that were bringing blood flow to the AVM have been cauterized or clipped and then divided. The AVM is now collapsed down and is only attached to the brain by the veins that previously drained the blood away from the malformation. The surgeon then clips and divides the veins. The AVM is finally free. The brain tissue is then carefully checked to make sure no AVM tissue has been left behind, and that all bleeding points have been properly secured.

The dura is closed. The skull is replaced with metal plates, wire, or suture. The scalp is closed with suture as well. A sterile dressing is applied. The patient is allowed to awaken gradually. It is important that the blood pressure be controlled carefully for the first day or two after surgery, so most people spend at least 24 hours in the intensive care unit after this type of operation. If all goes well, the person will awaken without any new problem and can expect to stay in the hospital for anywhere from 3 days to a week.

Like any surgery, the removal of a brain AVM carries certain risks. These include infection, bleeding during or after the surgery, brain injury, and even death. Obviously, surgery also carries the usual risks of being under a general anesthetic. Infection or bleeding after the operation may be minor problems or, in severe cases, may require further surgery. Brain injury may cause weakness or paralysis, numbness, speech difficulty, vision loss, or any other loss of brain function. This may be temporary, resolving to a variable extent with time and rehabilitation, or may be permanent. The risk of a major complication from surgery will vary depending on the size and location of the AVM and the skill of the surgeon.

In general, small AVMs in non-critical parts of the brain should carry a major complication rate well below 5%. The risk for larger AVMs may be 10% or greater, and very large AVMs may carry complication rates of 25% or more. The main point is that surgery for removal of an AVM should be performed only when the surgeon feels that the risk to the patient is justified by a greater risk of leaving the AVM untreated. This will be discussed below in the section on treatment recommendations.

Bleeding during the surgery may result from the AVM itself or from a phenomenon known as "normal perfusion pressure breakthrough". This is a rare phenomenon, but when it does occur, it may be a fatal problem. As you may recall from our discussion of "vascular steal" in the last chapter, an AVM may deprive the surrounding brain of normal blood supply. In these cases, the small arteries bringing blood flow to the brain around an AVM aren't used to carrying the normal amount of blood flow. When an AVM is removed, all of a sudden, these small arteries suddenly receive a large amount of blood supply, blood that was previously going through the AVM. In rare cases, the small arteries may not be able to tolerate the new increased pressure. The arteries can rupture, resulting in severe bleeding and swelling in the brain around the AVM.

This is called normal perfusion pressure breakthrough because the arteries are rupturing or experiencing "breakthrough", despite the fact that they are receiving blood flow under "normal pressure". The problem is that normal pressure is much more pressure than they usually face. This is also one reason why embolization may be useful to gradually shut down the blood flow through a large AVM prior to its removal. This allows the neighboring brain tissue to gradually acclimate to the new, increased (but normal) pressure as the flow through the AVM is gradually shut off.

Radiosurgery

Most people are familiar with the use of radiation to treat cancer. Radiation works by killing dividing cells. Since cancer cells are dividing at a much higher rate than normal cells, radiation therapy kills cancer cells but tends to spare the nearby normal cells which are dividing much more slowly. Many people don't know that radiation also kills tumors by killing the blood vessels that bring the blood supply to the cancer cells. As it turns out, high dose radiation will cause arteries to block off by damaging the cells in the walls of the arteries. The injured cells start to grow and then block off the lumen of the artery, the channel inside the artery through which the blood normally flows.

Today, high dose, focused-beam radiation is used commonly to treat AVMs of the brain. The radiation must be delivered as a high dose to work, and the beam must be perfectly focused so that it targets the AVM but doesn't injure the surrounding normal brain. The technique used to deliver this high dose, focused radiation therapy to brain AVMs is known as "stereotactic radiosurgery". It isn't really surgery, and no incision is required for the procedure. The technique utilizes stereotaxis or three-dimensional, computer localization to assist with the planning and delivery of the radiation.

The patient typically comes to the hospital the morning of the procedure. A "head frame" which looks like an open cage, is then attached to the skull. With the head frame in place, a CT scan or MRI scan and then an angiogram are performed. The head frame which remains fixed to the skull during these studies allows a computer to generate a three-dimensional model of the brain and the AVM in relation to the rigid frame. This means that the data from the scans and the angiogram can be entered into the computer and used to plan the radiation treatment.

Sophisticated software programs allow the computer to reconstruct the patient's brain along with the AVM in a three-dimensional model. This then allows the neurosurgeon to plan the dosing and route of radiation delivery. The planning phase typically takes a few hours during which time the patient can relax before the radiation treatment. Once the planning is completed, the radiation is delivered. This usually takes just a few minutes. Afterwards, the head frame is removed. The patient may be admitted to the hospital overnight for observation or may be discharged home. In most cases, only a single dose of radiation is all that is given.

Typically, the head frame is secured to the skull with four sterile pins that are attached directly to the skull bone after the scalp is numbed up with local anesthetic. Newer techniques use head frames that are designed with bite blocks to fit the patient's teeth. This type of frame is used in certain cases when the radiation is going to be delivered over multiple different days. This may be chosen when the AVM is located next to a very critical part of the brain such as the brainstem. Using multiple "fractions" of radiation, i.e. delivering the radiation in multiple treatments over different days, allows the surgeon to deliver a higher dose to the AVM while reducing the risk of injury to the nearby brain tissue.

There are two basic methods that are available for the delivery of stereotactic radiosurgery. The first is known as the "gamma knife", the other is the "linear accelerator". There is some debate among neurosurgeons over which technique is better, gamma knife or linear accelerator. Each seems to have some advantages and disadvantages, and each has its strong proponents. From the author's perspective, the individual performing the procedure, whether it be gamma knife or linear accelerator, is much more important than which technique is used. There are very good, very competent neurosurgeons who use each technique, and the patient is best off when they are treated by an individual with expertise in the management of AVMs no matter which specific device is used to deliver the radiation.

What are the risks of radiosurgery? Most people know that radiation can be dangerous. Anytime radiation is delivered to any part of the body, some normal cells will be killed. No technique is so precise as to allow delivery of radiation only to the abnormal area without exposing the normal surrounding tissue to a small amount of radiation. "Radiation necrosis" is a term used to describe the necrosis or injury of normal brain tissue around the AVM, the true target of the radiation. Using current technology, the risk of radiation injury to the brain from radiosurgery should be less than 3%. If radiation injury does occur, it can result in progressive neurologic dysfunction causing weakness or paralysis, numbness, speech trouble, visual loss, etc. Radiation injury typically appears between 6 months and 2 years after the radiosurgery is performed. It may be very difficult to treat this type of radiation injury, if it does occur.

One important point about radiosurgery is that it works slowly to cause the AVM to obliterate. After the radiation is given, it may take two, three, or even four years for an AVM to disappear. This means that there is some risk of bleeding while the radiation is working, until the AVM is occluded fully. In addition, not all AVMs respond to the radiation. It appears that small AVMs will respond in a high percentage of cases (80–90%), but not in every instance. Larger AVMs may respond in only 40–60% of instances, and very large malformations will rarely disappear after radiosurgery. Consultation with an expert in this area is strongly recommended to assess the likelihood that radiosurgery will successfully obliterate a particular AVM.

Medical palliation

We have already discussed the concept of palliation in the section on embolization. As mentioned above, some AVMs are not treatable using the conventional measures available to us today. They may be too large for radiosurgery to work and so big that surgery would almost certainly cause severe, irreversible neurological deficit. In these cases, embolization may be useful to improve the patient's symptoms. In addition, antiseizure medicines are important if seizures are a problem for the patient. Also, a number of antiswelling medications may be used to decreased the swelling of the brain around an AVM. These medications are rarely used any more because improving technology has increased our abilities to use surgery, radiosurgery, and embolization to treat more difficult AVMs or at least to reduce their symptoms.

Treatment Recommendations

Deciding which treatment is best for a given patient may be relatively straightforward or very difficult. Examining some "extreme" examples may be helpful in illustrating this point.

Imagine an eighty year-old man who is involved in a car accident and is found to have a large AVM in a critical area of the brain on a CT scan. The AVM is an incidental finding and is not causing symptoms. Furthermore, the risk of the AVM causing symptoms during the patient's anticipated life expectancy is very low. The AVM is large and in a critical location. This means that radiation will probably not be effective and surgery will carry significant risk of hurting the person. Embolization alone would be unlikely to cure the AVM and might cause a stroke. Given these points, any attempt at treatment would probably be a mistake. Observation alone is clearly the best treatment in this setting.

At the other extreme, imagine a small AVM that has bled three times in the past year and that is located in a non-critical area of the brain of a 15 year-old boy. The AVM has bled multiple times already and is likely to bleed again. Observation alone would not be reasonable given the young age of the patient. Radiosurgery might work well in this case, but would probably take at least two years to obliterate the AVM. Given the small size and the favorable location of the AVM, surgery would offer the potential for a rapid cure in this case and would represent the best treatment option. Embolization might be used before surgery or might not be necessary.

As a final case, imagine a 35 year-old woman with seizures resulting from a small AVM located right in the "speech area" of the brain, the part that allows the person to talk. The AVM has never bled. Given the young age of the patient and the fact that the AVM is causing symptoms, some treatment is probably appropriate. Because the AVM is located right in the speech area, surgery could cause permanent or at least temporary difficulty with language function for the patient. This would be a very reasonable case for radiosurgery which has a high likelihood of obliterating the small AVM over time and might be safer than open surgery. The likelihood of bleeding is low during the 2 to 3 year time interval before the AVM disappears. The patient can be treated with anti-seizure medications as well.

These are relatively straightforward examples. Unfortunately, most cases are not so simple for the surgeon. A number of general principles may be useful as guidelines.

First of all, AVMs that have bled repeatedly should be treated in the vast majority of cases to prevent further bleeding. If surgery is feasible, this would be the recommended treatment because radiosurgery will take several years to work, and during this interval, the patient could bleed again. If surgery is considered too dangerous, for example, if the AVM is in the center of the brainstem, then radiosurgery should be performed. At the other end of the spectrum, AVMs that are discovered by accident should be considered for treatment only if the patient is reasonably young, in good health, and treatment can be performed with reasonable safety and efficacy. The ultimate decision will depend heavily on the particular experience of the neurosurgeon.

Certain anatomic features of the AVM as defined on the arteriogram may be useful in deciding on the appropriate management of an AVM. As already mentioned, the size and location of the AVM in the brain will determine the safety of surgical therapy for the AVM. In addition, the arteriogram may reveal a narrowing of the vein that drains the blood flow away from the AVM. This might indicate an increased risk of future bleeding since the exit pathway for blood from the AVM may be partially closed raising the pressure in the AVM. This finding may argue for a more aggressive course of therapy. In addition, the presence of aneurysms associated with the AVM may increase the danger of leaving the AVM untreated, and this must be weighed into the decision-making process.

Patients who are having symptoms from an AVM are generally considered for treatment. If the AVM is small and in a location that is favorable for surgery, then this is typically the preferred treatment option. If surgery goes well, the patient is cured of the disorder and is unlikely to have a problem from the AVM in the future. If the AVM is small but in a very dangerous location for surgery (for example if it situated in the brain right next to a critical area), then radiosurgery is a reasonable choice. It has a high likelihood of obliterating a small AVM and carries less of a risk to the neighboring brain tissue than surgery.

If the AVM is medium-sized, then surgery becomes more attractive if feasible because radiosurgery is less likely to be effective. Nevertheless, if the surgeon feels that open surgery is likely to cause a major disability, then radiosurgery may be considered in this setting. If the AVM is large or giant, then radiosurgery is unlikely to be useful. Surgery can be performed but is more dangerous and should only be considered if the AVM bleeds repeatedly or causes progressive severe symptoms. Embolization may be useful in this situation as described above. No treatment may be the best option for most of these patients.

As mentioned above, after an AVM bleeds, we typically wait one to two months before proceeding with surgical removal of the AVM. Immediately after the bleeding, the brain tends to be swollen, and if the surgery can be deferred for several weeks, then the operation is likely to be better tolerated by the patient. In cases where a large blood clot is putting significant pressure on the brain, immediate surgical removal of the blood clot may be necessary. In general, if the clot can be removed without causing bleeding from the AVM, then the clot should be removed but the AVM left alone. Delayed surgery can then be performed under more controlled circumstances. If the AVM is very small, in a very superficial location on the surface of the brain without a deep component, or if the AVM ruptures during the surgery, then the AVM may be removed at the same time as the blood clot.

One important point in regard to this is that immediately after an AVM bleeds, the person may have a significant but largely reversible neurologic deficit. In other words, left alone, even a complete paralysis or other severe disability may fully recover as the blood clot is reabsorbed by the body. In the past, some surgeons have rushed in and removed the AVM while the person is in poor condition. In this setting, the person is left with a permanent paralysis because of the surgery that might have recovered if nothing had been done. This is unfair to the patient. It is more appropriate to wait several months, see if the patient recovers, and then decide on the safest treatment option. Surgery may not be a reasonable option at this point if it will likely cause a permanent disability. Radiosurgery may be a better choice in this situation.

It should be noted that the reason we can wait before going ahead with surgery in the case of an AVM is because after an AVM bleeds, the risk of rebleeding from the AVM is only slightly increased, possibly rising to twice the baseline risk of bleeding over the following six months. So if the risk of bleeding is normally 1% to 3% per year, it may increase to as high as 6% for the six months after the bleed. Then the risk returns to its baseline. In contrast, once an aneurysm bleeds, the risk of rebleeding is increased to greater than 40% over the six months after the bleeding, and we cannot "afford" to wait a few weeks, because the risk of fatal rebleeding during those weeks is too high.

When aneurysms are found in association with an AVM, the treatment becomes even more complicated. Each case is so unique that it is difficult to outline specific guidelines for the management of this situation. It should be mentioned that small aneurysms located on the large arteries carrying blood flow to the AVM may actually shrink down and disappear over months to years after the AVM is removed. The aneurysms in these cases are most likely related to the increased flow through the arteries carrying blood flow to the AVM. Once the AVM is gone, the flow is reduced, and the aneurysms can regress spontaneously. Larger aneurysms are unlikely to disappear and may require separate treatment. Again consultation with an experienced cerebrovascular neurosurgeon is strongly recommended in this setting.

In summary, each case must be carefully evaluated by an experienced neurosurgeon. This is a very complex subject, and AVMs are rare enough that they should be treated by neurosurgeons with expertise in their management. These general guidelines are meant only to give the reader a feeling for the factors that go into the decision-making process when evaluating the patient with an AVM.

CHAPTER 10

Cavernous Malformations of the Brain

What is a Cavernous Malformation?

A cavernous malformation is a particular type of vascular malformation of the brain. As described briefly in Chapter 7, cavernous malformations are small clusters of abnormal, thin-walled blood vessels that can occur anywhere within the substance of the brain. When removed at the time of surgery or at autopsy, the cavernous malformation resembles a tight cluster of small, darkly colored grapes. Alternatively, cavernous malformations are often said to look like mulberries.

The normal brain contains multiple arteries, capillaries, and veins running through the tissue of the brain to supply and then drain away blood flow, rich in critical oxygen and nutrients. AVMs, venous angiomas, and capillary telangiectasias are characterized by abnormally developed blood vessels that are running through brain tissue. Cavernous malformations are different from other vascular malformations in that there is no normal brain tissue located between the abnormal vessels of a cavernous malformation. The cavernous malformation is a densely packed collection of vessels that sit, like a compact ball, inside the surrounding, normal brain. This point becomes important when we think about surgery to remove a cavernous malformation, because if we can reach the malformation safely (i.e. without going through critical brain tissue), then the malformation can be removed without causing injury to the brain.

Why Do Cavernous Malformations Develop?

We don't know why cavernous malformations form. In certain individuals, a specific genetic abnormality involving the seventh chromosome has been linked to the development of cavernous malformations. We don't understand what function the gene in this location controls. It probably has something to do with the normal development of brain arteries, and research efforts are actively underway to examine this question. The more we understand about what goes wrong in the brain that allows a cavernous malformation to form, the more likely we will be to figure out how to prevent this process. The strong genetic basis for the development of cavernous malformations is further discussed below in the section on multiple lesions which often run in families.

As discussed in Chapter 7, the majority of vascular malformations appear to occur on a congenital basis and are probably present at birth. Interestingly, it is well established that cavernous malformations can develop in areas of the brain that were clearly normal in the past. Although most people with cavernous malformations have no known predisposing factors, environmental influences such as radiation exposure, can cause the formation of a cavernous malformation. Patients treated with radiation therapy for a brain tumor or leukemia have clearly been shown to develop new cavernous malformations that were not present on previous scans of the brain. The significance of environmental influences in this setting is also a topic of active investigation by medical researchers.

How are Cavernous Malformations Diagnosed?

Cavernous malformations have a tendency to bleed repeatedly into themselves. Typically, these are "microhemorrhages" in which the bleeding is entirely contained within the confines of the lesion itself. The cavernous malformation seems to have a well-developed capsule (outer wall). In addition, blood flowing inside the cavernous malformation seems to be under very low pressure. Because of the thick capsule and the low-pressure blood flow inside the cavernous malformation, the bleeding rarely breaks through this capsule. This is in distinction to AVMs, which, as you will recall, typically cause significant bleeding into the surrounding brain tissue, well outside the boundaries of the AVMs themselves. Remember that blood flowing in an AVM is under very high pressure, the same pressure as in any other large size artery of the brain.

Each time a cavernous malformation bleeds into itself, it tends to enlarge. If nothing is done surgically, the blood within the cavernous malformation will gradually break down, and some of it will be reabsorbed naturally by the body. Because of this, a cavernous malformation may change in size depending on whether it has undergone recent bleeding. Immediately after a hemorrhage, the cavernous malformation will be larger. As the blood reabsorbs, the malformation will shrink to some degree. Nevertheless, not all the blood tends to be reabsorbed by the brain, and the repeated hemorrhages tend to cause the cavernous malformation to enlarge gradually over time, growing a bit with each hemorrhage.

Cavernous malformations come to medical attention in one way or another because of these repeated hemorrhages. The bleeding can cause seizures or headaches or loss of neurological function. Seizures have already been discussed in several sections of this book. You may remember that a seizure results from a sudden burst of electrical activity within the brain. This electrical activity comes from an abnormal area of the brain that is irritated and overly excitable for some reason. After an aneurysm ruptures, the blood on the surface of the brain can irritate the brain and cause a seizure. AVMs can impair the normal blood flow to parts of the brain, causing the brain to become irritable and resulting in seizures.

Cavernous malformations, especially when they bleed, can irritate the surrounding brain because of the sudden expansion of the malformation itself or because of the blood products that are released by the malformation. Either of these can cause an increase in the local electrical activity of the brain, and this can produce a seizure. As described previously, a seizure can be a mild or a severe event. Some seizures are nothing more than staring spells, and it may not be obvious that the person is even having a seizure. A mild seizure may cause just a bit of numbness or tingling of an arm or leg. But if the electrical stimulation is large enough, the signal spreads throughout the brain, and the person may have a "full blown" seizure with loss of consciousness and violent shaking of the arms and legs. This is what most people think about when they hear the term "seizure". Anything ranging from a very mild to a grand-mal ("full blown") seizure may be caused by a cavernous malformation.

The bleeding from a cavernous malformation may cause nothing more than a severe headache. The headache typically results from a sudden, worse than usual hemorrhage in the malformation. Because the bleeding is contained within the malformation, headache may be the only manifestation of such a hemorrhage. Alternatively, bleeding into a cavernous malformation can cause sudden enlargement of the malformation, and if the malformation is located next to a part of the brain that controls an important function, the enlargement may result in neurologic dysfunction (weakness, numbness, speech difficulty, visual loss, etc.). The specific problem will depend on the specific location of the cavernous malformation. For example, if the malformation is located in the occipital lobe where vision is controlled, bleeding may result in a loss of vision.

Because the bleeding rarely escapes into the surrounding brain, any disability caused by bleeding from a cavernous malformation will usually recover, in large part, given time and rehabilitation. This will be discussed below in the next section. Rarely, a cavernous malformation may cause a severe hemorrhage, and this can be life-threatening. Alternatively, if the malformation is located in a particularly critical part of the brain, the bleeding can also be very dangerous (see below).

There is nothing particularly unique about the symptoms of a cavernous malformation that would allow for a definitive diagnosis without radiological studies. The sudden onset of headache, seizure, and/or neurologic disability may be caused by numerous different disorders. When a patient reports these or similar symptoms, the most useful radiological imaging tests are CT scan and MRI scan (see Chapter 2 for a full discussion). Cavernous malformations may be visible on CT scan, but their appearance is nonspecific. They are identified most easily on MRI scanning, and their appearance on MRI is highly specific. They show up as focal areas of abnormality, containing blood products of multiple ages because of the repeated hemorrhaging that occurs within them.

Interestingly, because the flow of blood within cavernous malformations is extremely sluggish, these lesions only rarely show up on routine angiograms. Remember that an angiogram is a test in which dye is injected directly into the arteries carrying blood flow to the brain. The contrast dye will fill the arteries, then the capillaries, and finally the veins of the brain. The more blood flowing in a particular malformation, the better it will show up on an angiogram. Cavernous malformations don't have much flow, so they don't show up well on an angiogram. Because of this, cavernous malformations are sometimes referred to as "angiographically occult malformations". Occult means hidden, and cavernous malformations may be "hidden" or invisible on an angiogram.

Finally, it should be mentioned that each time a cavernous malformation bleeds and causes a deficit (a neurologic disability), the patient tends to recover over time but is often left with a little bit of permanent weakness or numbness or vision loss or whatever other problem may have come on when the malformation bled. Therefore, the typical course of the patient with a cavernous malformation that bleeds repeatedly is one of very gradual loss of neurological dysfunction. Each time the malformation bleeds, assuming it's located near an important area of the brain, the person loses just a little more function.

Interestingly, before CT and MRI were available, some people who actually had cavernous malformations were misdiagnosed as having multiple sclerosis. Multiple sclerosis or MS is a disease of gradually progressive loss of neurologic function due to breakdown of the normal insulating material of the brain and spinal cord. Before doctors could visualize the presence of a cavernous malformation, individuals with these lesions were thought to have MS because of the similar stepwise progressive nature of the two disorders. Years later, when MRI became available, the cavernous malformations were discovered.

How Dangerous are Cavernous Malformations?

As already detailed, the blood flow within cavernous malformations tends to be sluggish and under low pressure. Because of this, they are relatively safer lesions in comparison with AVMs of the brain. Remember, cavernous malformations appear to bleed at a rate somewhere between 0.5% and 2% per year. This is relatively high. On the other hand, most of the hemorrhages are not symptomatic or result in only headache. Of those hemorrhages that do cause symptoms, the majority result in a seizure from which the person recovers fully or in the new onset of a disability which resolves significantly over time. It would be a mistake to consider cavernous malformations entirely "benign" lesions. Left alone, they can cause significant trouble. Nevertheless, they are not typically as dangerous as AVMs or brain aneurysms.

Also, it must be remembered that cavernous malformations can occasionally result in a severe hemorrhage. These rare cases may result in a life-threatening situation. If a cavernous malformation is located in a critical area of the brain such as the brainstem, the bleeding may also be very dangerous. The brainstem has so many important structures packed tightly together that any sudden enlargement of the malformation may result in sudden coma or irregularities of the heart rate, blood pressure, or breathing. This too can be a life-threatening situation. Therefore, rarely, cavernous malformations may be very dangerous lesions.

Can You Get More than One & Do they Run in Families?

Interestingly, a relatively high proportion of individuals with cavernous malformations have multiple malformations, and there is a strong predilection for this particular type of vascular malformation to run in families. Significant research has been devoted to studying these individuals and their families. This work has helped to identify the genetic basis of cavernous malformations as described above in this chapter. It should be mentioned that the familial form of cavernous malformations appears to be particularly prevalent in people of Hispanic descent. A large number of these families have been identified and followed in the Southwestern United States. If more than one individual in a family has a cavernous malformation, the rest of the family can be screened with MRI studies.

What are the Treatment Options for Cavernous Malformations?

As we have discussed in regard to every other problem in this book, the first option in the management of cavernous malformations is observation alone. This means that no direct intervention is performed, and the patient is followed over time to monitor the behavior of the malformation. As discussed above, for reasons that we don't understand, some cavernous malformations seem to have a tendency to bleed repeatedly while others may remain quiescent for prolonged periods of time. By waiting and watching, the patient and physician may gain an appreciation for how a particular cavernous malformation will behave over time. Repeated episodes of bleeding may argue for treatment even if the location poses some risk to the patient.

The second option in the treatment of a cavernous malformation is surgical removal. Cavernous malformations may be large or small and can be situated essentially anywhere within the substance of the brain. Because the blood flow within a cavernous malformation is under low pressure, it is unusual for the surgeon to encounter significant bleeding from a cavernous malformation during the operation. Therefore, the major determinant of the difficulty and risk of surgery is the location of the malformation within the brain.

The surgical removal of a cavernous malformation is typically performed with the patient asleep. The specific location of the scalp incision depends upon the location of the malformation. A small window is cut in the skull bone, and the dura mater (covering of the brain) is opened. At this point, the surgeon must enter the brain tissue over the malformation and work down to the malformation itself. Any tiny blood vessels that are bringing blood flow into the malformation are then cauterized and divided. By working 360 degrees around the circumference of the malformation, the lesion is freed from any attachment to the surrounding brain. It is then delivered as a single specimen.

Any residual bleeding is carefully stopped with electro-cautery. The skull is replaced with small titanium plates, wire, or suture. The scalp is closed. If surgery goes well, the patient typically spends one night in the intensive care unit (ICU). One or two days are spent on the floor recovering, and the patient is then discharged to home. If the cavernous malformation is located in a difficult location, the surgery may result in a new or worsening of an already present neurologic disability. For example, if the malformation is located in the back part of the right frontal lobe, right next to the area that controls motor function in the left arm and hand, the surgery may result in increased weakness of the left upper extremity. This will usually improve, but may require time and physical therapy.

Brief mention is made here of radiosurgery in the treatment of cavernous malformations. This subject has been discussed in detail in the chapter on AVMs. You may recall that high dose, focused beam radiation therapy as delivered by the gamma knife or linear accelerator has proven useful in the treatment of AVMs of the brain. Currently, there is no solid evidence that radiosurgery can cure a cavernous malformation. Nevertheless, some neurosurgeons have begun to use radiosurgery to treat cavernous malformations. Sometimes, the risk of surgery is very high, and it is hoped that the radiation will offer some decrease in the risk of future hemorrhage.

Unfortunately, follow-up MRI studies in patients treated with radiosurgery for cavernous malformations have not shown the malformations to shrink or disappear. Some neurosurgeons claim that patients treated with radiosurgery have experienced a decrease in the number of hemorrhages that they would have otherwise been expected to suffer. At this point, it is difficult to recommend radiosurgery for cavernous malformations because there is no evidence that it works, and there are risks associated with its use. In addition, even cavernous malformations in very delicate locations can usually be removed with low risk by surgeons who have significant expertise with this type of operation. Based on our current knowledge, only in very rare cases when some treatment is strongly recommended but surgery does not appear to be an option, would radiosurgery be considered as a treatment option.

What Treatment is Best for a Cavernous Malformation?

As with all conditions discussed in this book, it is difficult to make generalized recommendations about a problem that requires considerable individualized evaluation.

Nevertheless, some general guidelines can be given regarding the management of cavernous malformations. As already described, the management of these lesions may include observation alone, surgical removal, and rarely, radiation therapy.

For convenience, we can divide patients based on whether they have symptoms from the malformation or not. When a cavernous malformation is discovered by accident on a CT or MRI scan obtained for an unrelated reason (for example, if a scan is performed because the person was involved in a car accident), serious consideration may be given to following the lesion without treatment.

Only if the person is in excellent health, is reasonably young, and the lesion is located in a very safe location for surgery would surgical removal be recommended in this setting.

If a patient develops symptoms from a cavernous malformation, the specific symptoms and the surgical difficulty associated with removal of the malformation must be taken into consideration when making a treatment recommendation. In general, patients who are in good health and develop symptoms from a cavernous malformation that is located in a favorable (low risk) location for surgery represent the best surgical candidates. In this setting, if the cavernous malformation can be removed successfully, the patient is essentially cured and can get on with his/her life. On the other hand, if the risk of causing a permanent deficit with surgery is high, then the specific symptoms become more important in the decision process.

If a deep-seated, surgically inaccessible (i.e. difficult to remove with surgery) cavernous malformation is discovered because of seizures, and if the seizures are the persons' main concern, then anti-seizure medicines may be able to fully control the seizure activity and may be a reasonable treatment option (at least as a start). If the seizures are fully controlled with medicine, and the patient is not particularly worried about the **unlikely** risk of a severe hemorrhage, then it may be reasonable to follow things along with repeat MRI scans at regular intervals (say once a year), as long as no new symptoms develop. If this cavernous malformation remains stable on the yearly MRI scans, and the seizures are well controlled, then no further treatment may be required. Nevertheless, if the malformation then bleeds several times and/or if the repeat MRI in a year shows that the malformation has now enlarged because of repeated "micro-hemorrhages", surgical treatment must be reconsidered.

Brief mention is appropriate here of the management of cavernous malformations located in the brainstem. This is one of the most difficult areas of the brain to reach safely with a surgical procedure. The risk of causing new disability with surgery is higher in this location because so many important structures are packed into a small area inside the brainstem. Traditionally, cavernous malformations inside the brainstem have been considered "inoperable". In fact, recent work from a number of centers around the United States has shown promising results with surgery for cavernous malformations in the brainstem. Most authorities will only operate if the malformation has bled several times, proving that it will likely continue to bleed in the future.

It is critical that this type of surgery not be performed by an inexperienced neurosurgeon. The patient with a cavernous malformation of the brainstem should specifically ask any neurosurgeon who offers them surgery exactly how many of these operations (specifically in the brainstem) they have performed, and what their results have been. Only one or two of the most experienced surgeons in the world have performed 100 such operations. The majority of neurosurgeons have never operated on a cavernous malformation in the brainstem. This type of surgery should only be done in a center with dedicated expertise in this particular area.

Finally, as already mentioned, radiosurgery represents a theoretical treatment option for cavernous malformations. The benefit of radiosurgery has not been proven in any meaningful study. The reader should be aware that there are some neurosurgeons who use radiosurgery frequently in the treatment of cavernous malformations. Some are reputable individuals who feel strongly that "it works". In the author's practice, patients with cavernous malformations that are causing symptoms are considered for treatment. If, after discussion with the patient, a decision is made to treat the malformation, then surgery is considered as the optimal treatment for this problem. If the author does not feel comfortable performing the surgery (for example if the cavernous malformation is located in a difficult part of the brainstem where the author has not operated before), then the patient is referred to one of the leading experts in the country for surgical consideration. Only if that neurosurgeon, despite their greater expertise, felt that they could not safely operate on the patient would radiosurgery be considered. Again, the reader should be aware that they may hear a very different opinion about radiosurgery for cavernous malformations from other individuals.

CHAPTER 11

Other Vascular Malformations of the Brain

This chapter is devoted to a discussion of the remaining vascular malformations that can be found in the brain. The chapter will focus on capillary telangiectasias and venous angiomas. These two entities are similar in that they almost never cause symptoms, and, based on our current knowledge, they are present from birth.

Capillary Telangiectasia

A capillary telangiectasia, as defined in chapter 7, is a tiny aberrant collection of blood vessels, frequently found within the brainstem. Going back to Chapter 1, you may recall the story about Mr. Johnson's house. Remember there were pipes that carried the fresh water to his house and other pipes that carried the dirty water back to the plant. In the body, the arteries carry the blood from the heart to the brain, and after the brain has taken up the oxygen and nutrients from this blood, the veins carry the blood back to the heart again.

But as we discussed in the sections on AVMs of the brain, the arteries do not normally connect up directly to the veins. Rather, the arteries branch repeatedly, dividing into smaller arteries, then even smaller arteries called arterioles. Each time the arteries branch, they divide into smaller caliber vessels. Finally the arterioles empty their blood flow into very thin-walled vessels known as capillaries.

A capillary telangiectasia is a small collection of these tiny capillary vessels that forms inappropriately within the substance of the brain. These are typically tiny malformations, often just a fraction of a centimeter. In fact, the vast majority of capillary telangiectasias are found by accident and only at the time of autopsy. They almost never seem to bleed, and most are too small to be seen even on a good quality MRI scan. Therefore, there isn't very much to say about this entity. Capillary telangiectasias are almost never important from a medical perspective.

In chapter 8, we discussed extensively AVMs of the brain. Although the source of bleeding may be obvious in many cases of bleeding into the brain (aneurysm, AVM, or high blood pressure), there are a fair number of patients who have bleeding inside the brain with no identifiable cause for the bleeding. In these cases, MRI scanning and an arteriogram are performed but fail to reveal a source for the bleeding. In fact, it is possible that some of these patients may have very small AVMs that are just too small to see on these tests. It is also possible that some of these people may have capillary telangiectasias that have bled. Nevertheless, this possibility has not been proven, and from a practical perspective, capillary telangiectasias should be considered totally benign, incidental findings. They are often located deep within a portion of the brainstem known as the pons. This area is very difficult to reach with surgery, and surgical removal should not be performed. In almost all cases, capillary telangiectasias should be left alone.

Venous Angioma—Developmental Venous Anomaly

Venous angiomas are very common vascular malformations of the brain. The exact nature of these lesions has been clarified significantly over the past decade, and this has had major implications on our understanding of how they behave and how they should be treated. A venous angioma is also known as a developmental venous anomaly (DVA). This is probably a much better name because venous angiomas represent nothing more than unusual or anomalous patterns of venous drainage within the substance of the brain.

Normally, the arteries bring blood flow to the brain, branch repeatedly into smaller arteries, and eventually empty into the capillaries. The capillaries allow the blood to deliver oxygen to the brain, and then the blood flows on into tiny veins (venules) which join up with other tiny veins to become larger veins which keep joining with other veins until they empty into the very large veins which carry the blood flow out of the skull to reach the jugular veins on the way back to the heart.

Venous angiomas or DVAs appear to be "congenital anomalies". In other words, people are born with them. No two individuals have veins that develop in exactly the same way, and people with venous angiomas simply have an unusual variant in which multiple smaller veins (rather than joining with other small veins) empty directly into a large central vein which then travels through the brain tissue to reach the surface of the brain. This characteristic pattern is easily recognized on MRI scanning or with an angiogram. Because the multiple small veins draining into the angioma form a radial or circular pattern, the appearance of the venous angioma has traditionally been described as a "spoke-and-wheel" pattern or a "caput medusa" after the snake-filled head of the Greek Medusa.

It is critical to understand that these are essentially normal veins that happen to have formed in a funny pattern. These veins are essential to the normal functioning of the brain in that they are absolutely necessary to allow the blood that is brought in by the arteries to proplerly drain back to the heart. Venous angiomas almost never cause symptoms. In very rare instances, it is possible that they may cause bleeding or seizures, but this is almost never the case. **They must be left alone!**

To remove a venous angioma with an open surgery would shut off the normal channels that are needed to allow the blood to leave the brain. This could result in a very dangerous situation. Let's go back one last time to Mr. Johnson's house. Imagine that he had put in the pipes that brought water from the plant to his house, but then ran out of money and couldn't put in the drainage pipes to bring the dirty water back from the house to the plant. What would have happened the first time he turned on his faucet? Water comes in, goes down the drain, but then has nowhere to go. This can't go on for very long before things start backing up. And then, once again, Mr. Johnson would be standing knee deep in water.

As you can imagine, if blood is flowing in and has no way of getting out, the patient is at high risk for bleeding into the brain. When the exit channels (veins) are gone, high back-pressure can build up in the arteries and capillaries. If the pressure gets high enough, it may be too much for the walls of the arteries and capillaries to tolerate, and then they can rupture.

As MRI has become increasingly common, we are finding more and more patients with venous angiomas. Some have headaches, some have other symptoms. What is clear is that in the vast majority of these cases, the venous angioma is entirely asymptomatic and incidental. Again, they must be left alone. Although, venous angiomas may be visible on a CT scan of the brain, they are much more easily recognized on MRI scanning. Because they represent important venous drainage channels, they are also easily visualized on a routine angiogram in which the dye can be seen flowing through the arteries and capillaries and then into the venous angioma as well as the normal veins in the other parts of the brain.

Under the rarest of circumstances, venous angiomas may produce symptoms. It is possible that one of the branches of the venous angioma may be injured or may clot off because there may be slightly higher flow than normal in the large branches of a venous angioma than is present in other normal veins. In these very rare cases, there may be seizures or even bleeding related to a venous angioma. Nevertheless, for all practical purposes, venous angiomas should be considered entirely benign. The reason that venous angiomas are much more important to doctors than capillary telangiectasias is that they're larger and so they are easily recognized on MRI. Therefore, we find them much more often, and the possibility arises that an unsophisticated surgeon may recommend their removal or treatment with radiation. As explained, this is a very serious mistake.

One final point should be made about venous angiomas. As mentioned briefly already, venous angiomas can occur in conjunction with other vascular malformations, particularly with cavernous malformations. The exact connection between the presence of these two distinct vascular malformations within the brain is uncertain. They are often attached to one another, with the cavernous malformation draining blood directly into one of the tributaries of the venous angioma. It is hard to imagine that their coexistence in these cases is merely a coincidence. What we don't know is whether their occurrence together represents a cause-and-effect relationship or an expression of an improperly formed collection of arteries and veins within the affected part of the brain.

Does the venous angioma somehow encourage the formation of the cavernous malformation? Did they both form together because of some basic genetic problem with the blood vessels of the brain? We don't know.

At the same time, it is worth noting, that prior to ten years ago, neurosurgeons and neurologists thought that venous angiomas were relatively dangerous lesions. It was believed incorrectly that venous angiomas carried a high risk of bleeding. Surgeons even removed venous angiomas to prevent them from bleeding. As already discussed, this often resulted in disaster. We now know that venous angiomas are often found in association with cavernous angiomas. We also know that cavernous malformations don't usually show up on an angiogram. Therefore, there were many cases in which patients presented with brain hemorrhages but whose angiograms showed only a venous angioma. In these cases, the venous angioma was presumed incorrectly to have been the source of bleeding, because it was almost impossible to diagnose the neighboring cavernous angioma, which was almost certainly the real culprit.

Today, we know that patients who have a brain hemorrhage and have a venous angioma on angiogram almost certainly have a cavernous angioma nearby, and that the bleeding was caused by the cavernous angioma. **If surgery is performed, we remove the**

blood clot along with the cavernous malformation, and we leave the venous angioma alone. This has proven to be a very successful treatment method in this particular setting.

GLOSSARY

Aneurysm—thin-walled blister on an artery at the base of brain. See Chapter 1 for detail.

Angiogram—diagnostic radiology study performed to search for an aneurysm or vascular malformation. The radiologist passes a catheter up from an artery in the groin to the arteries in the neck, then injects dye into the carotid and vertebral arteries while multiple x-rays are taken of the arteries of the brain.

Arteriogram—synonymous with angiogram

Artery—a thick-walled blood vessel carrying blood flow from the heart to any organ in the body including the brain.

Arteriovenous malformation (AVM)—a particular type of vascular malformation of the brain. An abnormal collection or tangle of arteries and veins located within the substance of the brain. AVMs appear to be associated with a maldevelopment of the small capillaries which normally connect the arteries and veins.

Balloon angioplasty—in the setting of severe vasospasm (see below), the neuroradiologist may perform an angiogram and then pass a catheter with a balloon on its tip all the way up into the narrowed brain artery, then inflate the balloon to mechanically dilate the artery.

Bypass—in rare cases when an aneurysm cannot be clipped or coiled, the surgeon may have to perform a bypass operation, bringing blood flow through a new channel beyond the aneurysm and then trapping the segment of the artery with the aneurysm between clips (see Chapter 3 for detail).

Capillary—small blood vessels that normally connect the arteries (which bring blood flow to the brain) to the veins (which carry the blood flow away from the brain). The capillaries are very thin-walled, allowing the blood cells to transfer oxygen and nutrients directly to the surrounding brain tissue.

Capillary telangiectasia—a particular type of vascular malformation of the brain. Typically located deep within the brain, this is a small abnormal collection of capillaries. They rarely (if ever) cause symptoms, and are usually found by accident at the time of an autopsy performed for an unrelated reason.

Cavernous malformation—also known as cavernous angioma or cavernoma. A particular type of vascular malformation of the brain. This is a compact collection of abnormal blood vessels that is located within the substance of the brain.

Clipping—the traditional surgical method for repairing an aneurysm in which the surgeon exposes the aneurysm and then places a metal clip that opens and closes like a clothespin across the base of the aneurysm so no more blood can enter the aneurysm (see Chapter 3)

Coiling—a newer treatment for aneurysms in which a neurosurgeon or neuroradiologist performs an angiogram and then passes a catheter all the way up into the skull to reach the aneurysm itself and then fills the aneurysm with fine platinum wire to cause the aneurysm to clot off.

Craniotomy—the generic term for all operations in which the skull is opened including the surgical procedure for clipping an aneurysm or removing a vascular malformation.

CT—abbreviation for CT scan or computed tomography scan. This is a special form of x-ray that is often the first test performed when aneurysm rupture is suspected. It is painless and is the best x-ray test to look for blood that has escaped after an aneurysm bleeds.

Embolization—a technique that may be used as part of the treatment of brain AVMs. This is performed by a neuroradiologist or a neurosurgeon. As an extension of an angiogram, a catheter is passed up into the arteries inside the brain, and the arteries supplying blood flow to the AVM are then blocked off from the inside with either glue or metal coils or a variety of other substances. This is often performed as a prelude to surgery, but occasionally, may be curative without additional therapy.

Endovascular—a generic term for treatment of an aneurysm or vascular malformation from inside the blood vessel. Aneurysm coiling and AVM embolization are examples of endovascular procedures.

Gamma knife—a device that is used to deliver high-dose, focused beam radiation for the treatment of AVMs (and also tumors) of the brain. This is one of two commonly used ways to perform radiosurgery.

GDC—short for Guglielmi Detachable Coils, the type of coils most typically used to treat aneurysms today.

Hydrocephalus—a generic term that describes too much fluid building up inside the brain. This may occur after aneurysm rupture or bleeding from an AVM and may be life-threatening. Emergency treatment with placement of a drainage tube to relieve the pressure may be required (see below –ventriculostomy).

Intracerebral hemorrhage—bleeding into the substance of the brain itself results in a blood clot or "intracerebral hemorrhage". "intra" means within, "cerebral" means brain, and "hemorrhage" means bleeding. This can result from bleeding within the brain from any cause including vascular malformations (such as AVMs or cavernous malformations) and high blood pressure.

Intraventricular hemorrhage—bleeding into the fluid-filled cavities in the center of the brain known as ventricles. Blood within the ventricles can impair the brain's ability to absorb the fluid normally. If the fluid builds up, this is known as hydrocephalus (water on the brain).

Linac (Linear accelerator)—a device that is used to deliver high-dose, focused beam radiation for the treatment of AVMs (and also tumors) of the brain. This is one of two commonly used ways to perform radiosurgery.

MRI—short for magnetic resonance imaging. This is a special radiology test that allows for excellent imaging of the brain. Para-doxically, MRI does not show up fresh blood as well as CT, so if bleeding from an aneurysm is suspected, CT is a better test.

MRA—short for magnetic resonance angiography, This test can detect most aneurysms and is often performed as a screening measure when an aneurysm is suspected.

Papaverine—a drug that causes blood vessels to dilate. In the set-ting of severe vasospasm, a neuroradiologist may perform an angiogram and then inject papaverine into the narrowed ar-teries to help them dilate.

Radiosurgery—the use of high-dose, focused beam radiation for the treatment of brain AVMs. This technique really doesn't involve open surgery, but is actually a specialized technique for targeting the AVM for irradiation while sparing the sur-rounding brain using computer guidance.

Subarachnoid hemorrhage (SAH)—bleeding into the space around the brain (the subarachnoid space). This occurs when an an-eurysm ruptures, but may also result from other causes of bleed-ing around the brain including a head injury from trauma (see Chapter 4 for details).

Vascular malformation—an abnormality in the development of the blood vessels within the brain resulting in an abnormal collection or pattern of blood vessels in the brain.

Vasospasm—Four to fourteen days after an aneurysm ruptures, the blood vessels at the base of the brain may develop spasm or narrowing. If severe, this can result in stroke. (see Chapter 4 for a detailed discussion).

Vein—a thin-walled blood vessel carrying blood flow away from an organ (in this book, the brain) and back toward the heart.

Venous angioma—also known as developmental venous anomaly. This is one type of vascular malformation of the brain. It rep-resents an unusual pattern of development of the veins in a particular part of the brain. Venous angiomas rarely cause symp-toms.

Ventriculostomy—a drainage tube inserted through a small hole in the skull into the fluid-filled spaces in the center of the brain to drain an abnormal build-up of fluid (hydrocephalus).

Wrapping—in rare cases when an aneurysm can't be clipped or coiled, the surgeon may choose to wrap the aneurysm with gauze material to promote scarring around the aneurysm wall and decrease the risk of future bleeding. (see Chapter 3).

Printed in the United States
5847

9 780738 837598